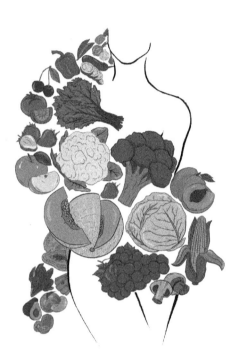

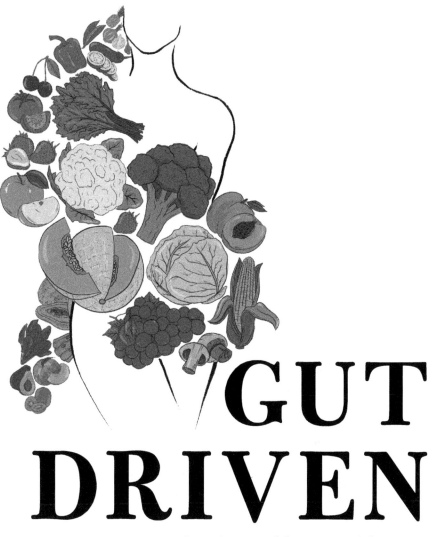

GUT DRIVEN

Jump-Start Digestive Health to Nourish
Body, Mind, and Spirit

ELLEN POSTOLOWSKI

Illustrations by Erin Hart

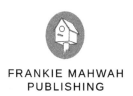

FRANKIE MAHWAH
PUBLISHING

Published by Frankie Mahwah Publishing, Allendale, New Jersey
www.chefellen.com

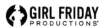

Edited and designed by Girl Friday Productions
www.girlfridayproductions.com

Cover design: Megan Katsanevakis
Interior design: Rachel Marek
Project management: Sara Spees Addicott
Editorial production: Jaye Whitney Debber

Illustrations by Erin Hart

ISBN (paperback): 979-8-218-05071-9
ISBN (e-book): 979-8-218-05072-6

*For my father, Frank Postolowski, who always told me,
"When you have your health, you are the richest person
in the world." You are always in my heart, Dad.*

CONTENTS

INTRODUCTION

Bloating. Sugar cravings. Migraines. Aggravated skin. Extra weight. Mood swings. Poor sleep. Perhaps you've struggled with these maladies for weeks, months, or even years. You know you can be doing better, but how? General practitioners claim you are fine, or maybe it's irritable bowel syndrome, or maybe the onset of lactose intolerance. Maybe.

You might have tried fad diets, ingested supplements, or gone keto. Trends like these may help in the short term, but they miss the mark on two fronts: they don't address the core problem that is going on, and they don't give you the know-how to design a lifelong eating regimen that supports your physical and mental well-being and is tailored to your unique digestive needs.

Gut Driven is your path to a healthier life, designed to jump-start your health from the gut up based on this philosophy: you are only as healthy as the food you can digest. When the gut is healthy, your hormones are balanced, your brain functions improve, and your immune response is prepared to defend your body against illness. We tend to ignore or medicate symptoms like gas, bloating, trouble sleeping, and cravings, but this kind of bandage doesn't address the root cause and can lead to chronic illness and even autoimmune disease.

It is possible to heal yourself, but if you change nothing, nothing will change. When you begin with an understanding of physiology and work on the fundamental cause of your illness, you build a strong foundation that you can rely on and maintain. My approach offers a practical, sustainable solution that targets the problem—what you eat and how you eat—rather than superficially addressing the symptoms. The bonus is that better gut health can enhance overall whole-body well-being. Wipe out unwanted inflammatory reactions, cravings, hunger, unexplained weight gain or loss, and food fear. Get back on your feet and experience the positive effects of a renewed attention to self-care and food. With proactive transformation comes confident choices, better sleep, more energy, improved cognitive function, and an overall desire to sustain the progress you've made.

Thank you for making this commitment. I am excited to be your guide on your journey to improved health. Let's get ready to reset!

MY GUT STORY

There's a saying: "You are not required to set yourself on fire to keep other people warm." How true this is! For me, not finding time for self-care cost me my health. As a private chef specializing in proper nutrition for my clients, I spent a lot of time caring for others, but that meant that I was often left behind. I ate well when I found the time, as a healthy lifestyle was my mantra, but the imbalance of many quick or skipped meals and stressful situations not handled properly eventually caught up to me. In order to truly embody that healthy-chef role model, I needed more quality time outside the physical daily grind of my occupation; the wear and tear of life as a chef prompted my need to reinvent and evolve. I turned to education, and several certifications in integrative nutrition shifted and refreshed the model I had established. My desire was to coach clients to understand the importance of nutrition and apply that knowledge to the food they ate. For me, integrative education and its core fundamentals linked whole-body wellness on and off the plate. Little did I know that I would be one of my first clients.

As I found my niche with gut and hormonal health, I was diagnosed with severe osteoporosis at the age of fifty-one. When a practitioner informs you that you have the bones of an eighty-year-old woman and your risk of fracture is very high, you suddenly feel very, very old. How could this happen to me? I was an advocate of healthy living, leading by example, or so I thought.

Through many doctor visits, I learned that in the United States, we treat acute and chronic illnesses similarly: with pills, injections, and limited one-on-one time with experts. This treatment approach conflicted with what I was learning in school, where the focus was on whole-body wellness, self-care, and most importantly, the connections that gut health has throughout the body.

I wanted to address, understand, and fix my problem. But the more questions I asked, the deeper I had to dig to comprehend my situation. Were there signs when I went back ten years into my routine blood work? Yes, the red flags for me were consistently low white blood cells, endometriosis, years of reflux, and an untamed candy addiction. In addition, not handling stressful situations well effectively added to the warning signs. Unfortunately for me, no one medically assessing my records through the years deemed these warning signs valid.

Chaos was beginning to unfold. The assessment from my doctors was an overall dysbiosis—a disruption to the equilibrium of the natural bacteria in my body. This imbalance was diagnosed as possible irritable bowel syndrome (IBS), inflammatory bowel disease (IBD), or small intestinal bacterial overgrowth (SIBO), meaning the ratio of good to bad bacteria in my gut was turning my overall health against me. Meals got very bland as I feared debilitating gas, pain, and discomfort almost every time I ate. I started a FODMAP diet, which focuses on eliminating short-chain carbohydrates that are resistant to digestion. Though a sound idea in principle, I was presented with a generic diet plan that made me feel as though the doctors didn't have time or didn't care to consider my individual situation. Being told to change everything, follow a completely new protocol, and then return in six months was confusing and did not offer support when I was uncertain about the guidelines, which was often. Physically, I was starting to feel better, but the restrictive plan took a toll on me mentally. After six months of rigorously adhering to the recommendations, the nutritional deficiencies were still a major concern and the stress of it all actually heightened many of my original debilitating symptoms. Though the concept was initially helpful, there was nothing sustainable about this plan.

Then my father passed away in April 2020 from complications of stomach cancer. For years, he had frequently complained of too much acid in his stomach, when most likely he *lacked* the vital acid needed to break down food efficiently. For his symptoms, my dad was given a bandage in the form of prescription and over-the-counter acid blockers. An overabundance of stomach acid equates to symptoms like chronic reflux, but acid blockers cause stomach acid to become more alkaline (see Alkaline versus Acidic), which impedes the function of the stomach. The acid blockers only took into account the symptoms; they didn't fix what was broken. Ultimately, I believe that being on and off these acid blockers for years is what escalated the situation and contributed to my father's death.

The book you're reading results from being beyond frustrated with medical issues that I—and many of my clients—could not get answers to. In search of clarity, I became a certified integrative nutritional chef and health coach. As a health coach, I emphasize the need to link doctors and patients and offer trusted and scientifically sound advice about optimizing health and enhancing well-being. This book is not meant to replace medical advice, though I do use many current educational studies that support science and the intricate functions of the human body. I believe that we should value the fact that we are as unique as the next person, and if quality time can be spent understanding what "healthy" means, positive changes unfold. By using this knowledge in conjunction with practitioners that support your individual journey and circumstances, chronic illness, obesity, and autoimmune issues can be curbed. By tapping into positive lifestyle changes, we improve both physical and mental weaknesses.

As a health-focused chef, I live by the well-known motto: "Let food be thy medicine." It is obvious that eating more fruits and vegetables is in your best interest, but simply knowing that is not enough. By embracing the connection between self-care, better choices, enhanced gut health, cognitive functions, and hormonal balance, we begin to heal. Plus, food inspires! It gives us the opportunity to create and gather in community to enjoy the flavors each season brings.

WHAT IS RESET 90/10?

Reset 90/10 is a comprehensive three-week program focused on eliminating inflammatory foods and acquiring awareness of whole-body wellness for body, mind, and spirit. Inflammation in the body can manifest in many different symptoms that we tend to ignore, don't recognize, or just live with until the impact is considerable. Inflammation is the body's way of communicating distress and can start with something as simple as eczema, acne, painful periods, or acid reflux. Convenience foods, preservatives, stress, and even improperly chewing food can wreak havoc on the gut and its vital functions. Over time, these common symptoms escalate and become significant triggers to chronic and autoimmune illnesses.

This common-sense, back-to-basics approach utilizes plant-based options to calm the gut lining, break unhealthy habits, increase energy, support immune and hormonal functions, and allow your body to digest food properly. By temporarily eliminating inflammatory foods, you will give your intestinal tract a break, allowing healing without pills, meds, powders, or elixirs. As you heal, your body begins to restore essential bacteria and experience enhanced immune health, better cognitive functions, and balanced hormones.

Reset 90/10 is designed to be flexible and forgiving. In fact, the 90/10 part represents the ideology that doing something "perfectly" 90 percent of the time and "imperfectly" the remaining 10 percent is the way we make real and consistent progress. Reset 90/10 understands that we're all human, and as long as we have a built-in safety net, we'll have a greater chance of bouncing back. The 10 percent safety net is your reminder that Reset favors progress, not perfection. With this framework, you can release old habits, establish new ones, and build a better whole-health foundation.

During Reset 90/10, you'll also examine lifestyle practices that may not be serving you, such as an unhealthy diet, excessive stress, self-medicating, and other coping mechanisms—if you sometimes polish off an entire package of Oreos, always have that extra glass of wine, consistently work too much, or often stay in bed all day long, I have strategies to support you! In addition, you'll learn about the proven connection between the gut and the brain and how to improve mental health through food. Making time for yourself is a self-care act that is worth the effort. Twenty-one days of baby steps add up to giant strides over time, and the benefits are enormous, especially in an age when convenience foods and the standard American diet may cause the decline of your health.

The Reset phase is followed by the Maintenance phase, during which you'll reintroduce eliminated foods one by one. As you become more in tune with your body, you will also focus on potential sensitivities and intolerances. The positive foundation you've built will help you recognize negative physical or emotional changes from foods and empower you to make decisions that will benefit your gut health and, therefore, your overall health.

Physical transformation requires a mental shift. You have the power to change when you embrace a positive attitude toward challenges. Altogether, this program offers a complete look at how food affects the body, and strategies to get the most out of what you eat and feel better doing it. With optimized blood flow, improved alkalinity, fewer inflammatory responses, and greater mental ease, you will establish a foundation for whole-body health built specifically for you, by you.

IS RESET 90/10 RIGHT FOR YOU?

Can you imagine?

- Losing weight simply by eliminating inflammation
- Eating foods and not burping
- Not being constipated
- Sleeping soundly throughout the night
- No more watery stools and constant cramping
- No more gas
- Not having a bloated stomach 24/7
- Not craving sugar and salt all the time
- Having clearer skin
- Getting rid of migraines
- No more heartburn
- No more food intolerances
- No more reoccurring illnesses
- No more moodiness

This sounds heavenly, right? It can be your reality. And although I know you're fired up to get started, you wouldn't set off on a twelve-mile hike without preparation and gear. On this journey to rid yourself of uncomfortable chronic conditions related to inflammation and an unhealthy gut, the supplies you'll need are *time*, *effort*, and *commitment*.

Time: Timing is everything. You will need to choose three consecutive weeks for the Reset phase, plus several weeks beyond that for the Maintenance phase. If travel, the holidays, or any event that impacts your ability to eat regularly are in your near future, you may be more successful if you postpone your start date. Also be sure to consider events that might take up time or impact your routine such as surgery, a demanding work project, or a remodel of your kitchen (which, of course, you'll need access to).

Effort: Your health is your responsibility. You will need to spend time planning, shopping for, prepping, and executing meals, as well as attending to self-care. Reading this book is part of that, and you should plan to stay engaged by reading each chapter—even if you think it does not apply to you. Beyond the food, you will also need to spend some introspective time considering your lifestyle and working toward improvements in areas that need more attention. Your responsibility to your health requires a reflection of potential "off the plate" stressors such as relationships, exercise, and spirituality. Your health is worth the effort!

Commitment: This program breaks old habits and establishes lifestyle modifications, and a large part of that is through eliminating inflammatory foods. So you must be willing to remove animal protein and alcohol from your diet for three weeks. Why? Because these (among a few other specific foods) could be highly inflammatory. If just the thought of not being able to eat cheese or have a drink after work has you stressed, wait till the time is right. Ultimately, I want you to nourish yourself and enjoy your food without guilt or shame, so you must bring the right mindset, meaning you have a true desire to make changes and are committed to following through on your goals.

HOW TO GET THE MOST OUT OF THIS BOOK

This book is designed to give you the tools to take charge of your health, and if you're here, it's time to rewrite your story with a strengthened definition of what "healthy" means to you. So, to get the most out of this book, you may find yourself skipping around, revisiting certain sections if your health status changes or to refresh yourself on the

Make a Promise to Yourself

The good news is that it's not too late! Our bodies are capable of healing when we give them a little TLC, awareness, and the education that Reset 90/10 offers. If you have decided that this program is for you, please make the following commitment to yourself.

I accept and agree to

- Be coachable under the guidelines of Reset 90/10
- Be open to fresh, whole plant-based foods and concepts
- Eat nourishing foods according to the guidance in this book
- Find time for myself
- Find a healthy balance between work and play
- Have an appreciation for the relationships in my life
- Listen to my body's wants and needs
- Eliminate the stressors in my life appropriately

concepts, or tailoring the program to your needs. It's really up to you. I also recommend reading with a highlighter or tabs so you can mark important passages for easy reference. Bottom line: the more you put into it, the better you will feel.

In part 1, you will learn all about the gut and its direct connection to the brain, why inflammation is so harmful to your body, how stress impacts digestion, and other fundamental processes. Please do not skip this part! Educating yourself on how the gut works and how Reset 90/10 is designed gives you a strong foundation to make wise choices.

In part 2, you will be guided through the three-week Reset program. After a chapter on preparation, there is a chapter focusing on each of the three weeks.

In part 3, you will enter the Maintenance phase, learning how to safely reintroduce foods you eliminated. You'll establish the eating regimen that's best for you, while factoring in various health considerations, allergies, and intolerances.

Finally, part 4 houses all the recipes, separated into Reset and Maintenance recipes. The Reset recipes carry you through mealtime for the first three weeks and can be used throughout your entire journey. The Maintenance recipes ease you back into eating a wider range of foods and teach you how to move beyond the program confidently.

My hope is that this guide empowers you to trust your gut. With the knowledge and tools I share, you'll become more in tune with your body and learn how to meet its nutritional needs. Begin with the mindset that nothing is perfect, but because your health matters, you will try your best as each day unfolds. Your dedication will help this new way of life become as routine as brushing your teeth—consistency is the secret to achieving the best possible outcome! Whole-body self-care is integrative, combining education, lifestyle changes, and more balanced meals that limit inflammatory foods. With this approach, it is possible to heal your gut, alleviate frustrating symptoms, and improve digestive health with gentle, empathetic, and knowledgeable instruction.

PART ONE

Foundations of Gut Health

Welcome to part 1. In this section, you will learn about the crucial functions of the gut and its connectivity to many of our vital functions. Imagine your gut as the communication center of your body. Our gut must be in tip-top operation to effectively keep us healthy, resilient, and fueled properly. Our immune system depends on the health of the gut to keep invaders out and maintain a sound stability within. Good guys must prevail over bad. When there is a breach, that well-oiled machine is compromised.

In this section, the reading material will come in quite handy as you start making positive changes and see and feel results. Often, we retain what speaks to us the most and make connections throughout the process with many "aha" moments.

CHAPTER 1

Laying the Groundwork

Our goal during Reset is for processed foods to lose their appeal. By adjusting how, when, what, and how much you eat, you can figure out what works for you over the long term. I promise you will be shocked when you just don't crave those bottomless bags of potato chips, cookies, or sugary treats anymore! Then, we naturally gravitate toward better choices that are void of the inflammatory ingredients that made us sick in the first place. Filling up on better foods heals your relationship with eating and helps you move away from unhealthy habits. As you build this stronger foundation, you won't feel guilty about a wild night out drinking, platter of nachos, or occasional sugar indulgence. You have a deep-rooted desire to live your healthiest life. If indulgence suits you here and there, it's no problem, because you have that strong foundation to return to. But you must establish the foundation first, and that's where the Reset 90/10 principles come in.

There are many reasons our American culture is so hooked on processed foods. We are always on the go, and quick-and-easy options allow us to get more done. We are also easily persuaded by the endless witty and clever slogans that are everywhere we turn. In addition, we must consider social and economic factors. Fresh fruits and vegetables are not always available to many, because they are too expensive or not even stocked in the nearby grocery stores. But whatever the reason, health problems begin surfacing when we load up on convenience foods, which rely on too much sugar, fat, cheaply made fillers, and salt as typical ingredients. These ultraprocessed foods are recognized by the reward center of our brains, leading to a craving or an addiction, only exacerbating the cycle.

A deeper understanding of nutritional density will hopefully help you analyze what's really on your plate. Wanting to make healthful changes will reward you as you build this solid infrastructure. Because of social and economic limitations, some people simply cannot change with an all-in mentality, so I encourage smaller steps, explore affordable alternatives, and educate to make possible even the smallest shift toward the road that leads to greener pastures.

THE RESET 90/10 PRINCIPLES

How many times have you heard something along the lines of "eat more fruits and vegetables" in discussions about healthy eating? No one can argue with this popular advice! However, I want to make an important point: no matter how many fruits and vegetables you consume, you are not going to benefit from their nutrients if your digestion is impaired. Optimal health requires efficient digestion and proper distribution. And efficient digestion starts with a balanced microbiome—only then can nutrients be properly absorbed.

This is why the first principle of Reset 90/10 is that *you're only as healthy as the food you can digest.* If you have bloating, constipation, acid reflex, cramping, or diarrhea, you likely have an unhealthy gut. But did you know that poor sleep, exhaustion, skin problems, weight gain, thinning hair, lack of concentration, and other ailments are symptoms too? By eliminating inflammatory foods, acidity, food fear, and stress, you can give your overworked gut a break. Then, the focus can be on bringing in more plant-based foods that are easily absorbed. You will be satiated with less and on your way to absorbing vital nutrients with optimal intestinal responses. You will find no processed or artificial ingredients, no added processed sugars, no preservatives, no hydrogenated oils, and no additives in this plan or the recipes in this book. Deciding not to let these kinds of ingredients into the kitchen is a challenge, but it's one of the smartest choices for a strong food foundation.

The second principle of Reset 90/10 is that *your relationship to food, as to life, should be fun and flexible.* I'm not asking you to strictly adhere to a diet or lifestyle. In fact, to do so goes against everything I believe in and advise to my clients. Rigid rules, even in the name of "healthy eating" or "clean eating," can lead to a dieting mindset, dieting behaviors, or in extreme cases, an eating disorder known as orthorexia nervosa, an obsession with healthy eating that's associated with restrictive behaviors. A preoccupation with weight, certain foods, and restrictions are warning signs that can snowball out of control and lead to negative emotional and physical complications.[1] So that you never forget, the very title of this program is a reminder to practice the concepts 90 percent of the time and use the remaining 10 percent to guiltlessly indulge if the mood or occasion presents itself.[2]

This lenient approach sets us up for success because when we don't allow for freedom and flexibility, we open the door for bingeing, out-of-control cravings, and consequent shame to come in and rule us. Letting yourself bend the rules occasionally will help keep you on the optimal path. Remember: the mental side of food and nutrition is just as important as the physical side. I'm not perfect, and I don't expect you to be. So just aim for 90 percent dedication and 10 percent down-time while in Reset.

The fun comes in when you open yourself up to experimenting with food. You don't have to like everything, but trying new fruits and vegetables or different cooking strategies is part of the process. A variety of plant-based foods keeps your metabolism at its most efficient and gives your taste buds an adventure! A Reset may not sound like fun, as change can be difficult. I suggest making this commitment not only for the obvious reason of optimal digestive processes, but for your hormones, which—as you'll see—*need you* to bring balance within. Increased intake of better choices and more self-care leads to better moods, sleep, digestion, and bone and blood health, just to name a few positive side effects. In short, more happy times lie ahead. Are you up for that?

By approaching the next three weeks with this mindset, you become your own laboratory, testing what works and what doesn't. This speaks to the third principle: *you will eventually design your own maintenance plan.* No, you don't have to count calories or weigh food. You don't have to become 100 percent plant-based either. You simply pay attention to your body's cues, understand how the gut works, incorporate strategies for mental health, and ultimately make choices that serve your own best interests.

REMOVE, REPLACE, REINOCULATE, AND REPAIR

The four *R*s protocol has been used effectively for years in functional medicine for gut healing and understanding inflammatory responses.[3] Here's a brief summary:

- *Remove* inflammatory foods and irritants like stress, which increase the likelihood of yeast overgrowth, parasites, and bad bacteria in the body.
- *Replace* with foods that support optimal digestive functions, digestive enzymes, and *sufficient* stomach acid, leading to enhanced nutrient distribution.
- *Reinoculate* balanced gut flora and continue the maintenance of better gut and immune health by supporting good bacteria with probiotic and prebiotic foods. Microbiome diversity is a vital component of health.
- *Repair* cells, intestinal structures, and inflammation damage to achieve sustainable gut, hormonal, immune, and cognitive functions.

I mention the four *R*s protocol because it works, and these ideas are the backbone of Reset 90/10. The *R*s don't necessarily work chronologically, as achieving optimal digestion is always a work in progress. Meds, food poisoning, or a virus can easily throw the body off, but harmony starts in the intestinal tract. Bouncing back from an ailment is feasible when you reshape your gut. Supporting a healthy GI tract and eliminating potential inflammatory response triggers becomes easier when you pay attention to the details that the four *R*s emphasize.

HOW DOES DIGESTION WORK?

Digestion is the process of turning the food we eat into energy. Food particles must be broken down efficiently and absorbed into the blood or delivered to cells for energy or for future functions such as thinking, moving, and growing. This is a functioning metabolism.[4] The digestive system, also referred to as the GI tract, is one long muscular tube that starts at the mouth and ends at the anus.[5] It has two essential functions: *digestion* and *elimination*.

Our body starts the process of digestion before food enters our mouths. When we are hungry, our body sends a message to the brain that it needs to eat. The brain then activates digestive enzymes to be released. We taste, chew, produce saliva, and break down the food into smaller particles ready to be swallowed.

Food is then delivered to the stomach, where it is churned with acidic gastric acids and digestive enzymes. Gastric acids (or hydrochloric acid, HCL) break down the food, and digestive enzymes split up the proteins. The process of breaking down foods varies depending on the macronutrient composition of those particular foods (fat, protein, or carbohydrate). For example, a meal higher in fat or protein takes longer to break down than one rich in carbohydrates. However, not all carbs are created equal. Complex, starchy carbs like potatoes, bananas, and whole grains take longer to digest and are better for overall digestion, good gut flora, and nutrient density. Compare that to a simple-carb-loaded, high-protein, high-fat Big Mac and side of fries. Proteins have much more complex chemical compositions, therefore the task of breaking down the proteins into the amino acids we require for long-lasting fuel takes longer. Fat also affects the rate of digestion. Our bodies typically store excess calories and inflammatory foods as triglycerides in fat cells—an emergency energy source as opposed to immediate fuel. A surplus of triglycerides (fat) in the blood contributes to hardening of the arteries, inflammation of the pancreas, obesity, diabetes, and increased storage of fat in the liver.

After food is broken down in the stomach, it is delivered to the small intestine, and assistance from the liver, pancreas, and gallbladder comes into play. These organs participate by releasing juices that further break down the food into manageable forms of vitamins, minerals, and waste. The nutrients from carbs, protein, and fats are then transported across the small intestine and into the bloodstream as energy.[6]

Food should be mostly digested as it makes its way to the large intestine. Indigestible foods are typically insoluble fibers. They keep the intestines clean and keep us full and regular. But soluble fibers aren't bad—plant-based sources are superfoods for the gut and stimulate the growth of beneficial bacteria strains.[7] Most fruits and vegetables contain both fibers and are essential for proper bowel movements and colon health.

After a time, indigestible foods eliminate through the anus as feces.

FOOD BECOMES ENERGY

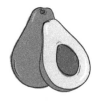

Everything is interconnected, and your gut is the epicenter. So let's look at how certain food groups get turned into nutrients through the process of digestion.

Fats: Fats need the chemical interaction of bile released from the gallbladder to create energy. Bile is stored in the gallbladder but must pass through the liver first, which plays a major role in how much fat is in your blood. Too much fat in the liver can damage it and keep it from doing its job. The liver is also responsible for the functions of cholesterol and triglycerides in our bodies. When broken down properly, cholesterol provides the bile needed to digest food. Triglycerides give us energy. In excess, these lipids are harmful and increase our risk for disease.[8] When our liver is sluggish, simple processes like creating energy, removing harmful toxins, making new blood, and utilizing nutrients are compromised. Recognizing the importance of dietary fat during Reset—and the time of day to ingest it—is a major step toward better wellness, so we'll discuss this more later as you plan your weekly menus in the Preparation chapter.

Protein: The breakdown of essential amino acids from proteins happens in the stomach. If you do not have adequate stomach acid or are bandaging acid reflux with meds, your stomach becomes more alkaline. This is great for relief, but relying on pills to cover up what could be a need for dietary improvements will cause that habitat to become too alkaline. Your gut environment must be highly acidic to break down foods and kill harmful bacteria. Physical and environmental stressors, such as surgeries, vitamin deficiencies, and age may also inhibit the production of vital acid.

Carbs: Carbohydrates are broken down by the release of insulin from the pancreas. When we do not have adequate digestive enzymes or sufficient insulin, the small intestine cannot completely process the nutrients as energy for the body.

SIGNS OF AN UNHEALTHY GUT

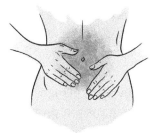

When your gut environment is healthy, you reap all the benefits of your food; when it isn't, you risk inflammation and ill health. If your body lacks digestive enzymes or adequate stomach acid, those molecules (from food) that provide energy, growth, and repair are compromised. Without proper enzymes and the optimal acidic environment, food goes undigested. This can lead to *dysbiosis*, an imbalance of the GI tract's microbiome, thought to contribute to a wide range of adverse health conditions, including reflux, gas, bloating, and leaky gut. These conditions make us vulnerable to chronic illness, hormonal and brain imbalances, and autoimmune disorders.[9]

Your gut also plays a role in regulating important hormones such as cortisol, serotonin, dopamine, and melatonin, thanks to the gut-brain connection, which you'll learn more about in Repair. For now, though, understand that an adverse gut-brain chemical reaction as a result of an imbalanced microbiome can lead to anxiety, excess weight, cravings, depression, sleepless nights, and dementia.[10]

As if that weren't troubling enough, an imbalanced gut can lead to food allergies, food sensitivities, or food intolerances (see Identifying Food Intolerances, Sensitivities, and Allergies). Ignoring warning signs and continuing to eat the wrong foods feeds the harmful bacteria and causes more inflammation. Inflammation is a signal to your body that something is wrong, so it sends help in the form of antibodies. When you are sick, this is exactly the response you want, but if it's happening constantly, it can alter immune responses and lead to disease. However, by reducing inflammation during the Reset phase, you can regulate hormones and help your gut, brain, liver, adrenal glands, and thyroid work properly again.

But what exactly is going on physically in your gut? The lining of your intestinal tract acts as a barrier between the intestine and the bloodstream. It is the most significant barrier against the external environment. So, as you might imagine, it needs to be resilient enough to knock out unwanted invaders (harmful bacteria) and toxins and protect the gut and immune system. When there is an imbalance of lifestyle choices and environmental factors, such as meds, stress, processed foods, poor diets, or traumas, our gut can become compromised. Let's look at some of the symptoms that may indicate an unhealthy gut.

High blood sugar levels: Processed ingredients and refined sugars can result in high blood sugar levels. Too little insulin or your body not using insulin properly is most often linked to diabetes. The medical term for high blood sugar is hyperglycemia. Symptoms may include imbalanced blood sugar levels, frequent urination, excessive thirst, rapid heartbeat, or vomiting.

Excess saturated fat: An overload of convenience foods and unhealthy fats creates an imbalance in the ratio of good to bad gut bacteria. Fatty foods can also destroy white blood cells, leading to an increased vulnerability of the gut lining and immune system. We all know too well when we have overindulged in a greasy meal. When this happens, the digestive process needs much more time to break down this food. In turn, you may feel nauseous, bloated, and uncomfortable. Long-term consumption of high-fat foods can raise "bad" LDL cholesterol and increase cardiovascular health issues.

Sweet and salty cravings: These cravings could indicate nutrient deficiencies. Is there an unlimited supply of gummies, Red Vines, or Swedish Fish in your home? There are no nutrients in these addictive processed snacks. Not all sugar is created equal, and the processed sugars in candies offer nothing but blood sugar spikes and crashes, which makes us crave them more. And then there are all the sugar substitutes that many people rely on to cut calories and excess sugar.

We become so hardwired by the chemicals and additives in processed foods that we don't realize that pathogens and harmful bacteria are thriving on these processed foods and sugars in our body.[11] Fruits and vegetables, on the other hand, provide natural sugar along with actual sustenance and other benefits.

Chronic fatigue or lack of quality sleep: When we are nutrient deficient because we are eating too many processed foods and not enough whole foods, our cells are not energized. Serotonin is an essential hormone that stabilizes our mood, increases feelings of well-being and happiness, and aids in sleep and digestion—and 95 percent of serotonin originates in our gut.[12]

Eczema, acne, and rosacea: Poor diets and food allergies or sensitivities may increase the risk of intestinal permeability. When harmful substances enter the bloodstream, it leads to inflammation and aggravated skin conditions.[13]

Weight gain or weight loss: An unhealthy gut can impair your body's ability to absorb nutrients, regulate blood sugar, and store fat. Weight loss can result from SIBO (too much harmful bacteria), while unintentional weight gain may result from insulin resistance or inflammatory responses.

The urge to overeat: This may be due to decreased nutrient absorption. You may be eating a "normal" amount of food, but if your gut is not breaking down foods properly and not providing that much-needed fuel, you become nutrient deficient. Our bodies want to correct, so we receive signals to nourish ourselves, but the cycle exacerbates the internal struggle and dysbiosis.

Migraines: Treating digestive symptoms can often lead to a reduction in the frequency and severity of migraines. When imbalances spiral out of control with something like a gluten sensitivity, celiac, or *H. pylori,* the associated widespread inflammation contributes to migraines.

Bloating or gas: When undigested foods sit and are not properly broken down in the small intestine, they ferment and release gases, which creates harmful conditions in an environment that does not thrive with an overabundance of bad bacteria.

Constipation: Too often, a lack of fiber or hydration constipates. Constipation is also linked with imbalances in good gut bacteria.

Suffering in this department leads to medications and over-the-counter relief. Unfortunately, some of these aids contain ingredients and additives that can further exacerbate the issue.

Recurring illnesses and autoimmune conditions: Consequences of an imbalanced gut include chronic UTIs and SIBO, Crohn's, fibromyalgia, Hashimoto's, Graves', and osteoporosis, to name a few.[14] These are more of the snowball effects of imbalances in the microbiome.

Food sensitivities: These can be the result of a compromised gut.[15] If there are issues with the intestinal structure, certain proteins are perceived as invaders. The body then releases antibodies to combat antigens. This is how food sensitivities start and spiral out of control.

A change in your poop: Feces are a good indicator of how healthy your gut bacteria is. Stool samples are used in functional medicine practices to help patients identify and hopefully correct an imbalance, for example, with elimination protocol, probiotics, or supplemental therapy. These tests can also specify an overabundance of yeast, changes in cell DNA, parasites, harmful infections, unbalanced pH, and too much fat in the blood.[16] The Bristol Stool Scale (see illustration), a chart that identifies seven types of stool consistencies, is an informative diagnostic tool for anyone with potential gastrointestinal maladies. I encourage all my clients to refer to this scale so they can be more conscious of how they eliminate, and then to relay this information to their practitioners.

Bristol Stool Scale

TYPE 1	TYPE 2	TYPE 3	TYPE 4
Separate Hard Lumps (Severe Constipation)	Lumpy and Sausage-like (Mild Constipation)	Sausage Shape With Cracks (Normal)	Like A Smooth Soft Sausage or Snake (Normal)

TYPE 5	TYPE 6	TYPE 7
Soft Blobs with Clear-Cut Edges (Lacking Fiber)	Mushy Consistency with Ragged Edges (Mild Diarrhea)	Liquid Consistency with No Solid Pieces (Severe Diarrhea)

EMPOWER YOURSELF

Let's not forget that *you* are a huge factor in making improvements to your gut health. Yes, you need the science, meal planning, and recipes to follow this program. But you also need to be your own advocate. Making the best choices with food on and off the plate starts this journey to heal and create the most optimal environment for health. If you are willing to heighten your awareness, balance will unfold.

I invite you to familiarize yourself with these six basic components of self-advocacy. Self-advocacy gets much attention in the workplace, but what if we applied some of those principals to protecting our well-being and the supportive building blocks we are now establishing? Now is the time to ditch the old habits and cultivate a willingness to learn and make better lifestyle choices. It's also the right time to find joy and balance and to let go of guilt, shame, and negativity. If you can be mindful of this self-advocacy approach while executing the protocol, you will succeed in this program.

1. *Believe in yourself.* Empowerment is about being adequately supported in every aspect of your life. As you become healthier, your confidence will grow. And with that, you'll develop a comfortable, progressive approach to making better food choices, establishing healthier habits, and cultivating stronger personal boundaries.

2. *Remember that prevention is early detection.* Preventive healthcare addresses potentially severe conditions before they become significantly harmful. This includes annual checkups, follow-ups, immunizations, and certain screenings.

3. *Seek balance.* Decide what you want or what needs to change. Are the physical, mental, emotional, and spiritual parts of your life in proportion to each other? If not, do you have a plan to control what's out of balance? When your health is off, don't count on others to make decisions. Concern yourself with all aspects of your health before moving forward after a prognosis.

4. *Get the facts.* Protect your rights and well-being. Be specific with doctors, arm yourself with information, keep records, and get a second opinion.

5. *Plan your strategy.* What is the best way for you to achieve your goals? If you have followed steps one through four, you should be well informed about many aspects of your well-being. Communicate and ask for help if you cannot advocate for yourself. There are resources and organizations to help you if you feel neglected or abused where your health is concerned.

6. *Be accountable.* Accountability is being responsible and proactive in all aspects of your well-being. You have a game plan, objectives, and goals. Take ownership of your choices and actions and don't blame others or make excuses.[17]

CHAPTER 2

Remove

The focus with eliminating foods is not to torture you, but rather to give you space to notice how not eating certain foods affects whatever issues you are dealing with. Three weeks is an optimal time span to calm the body, organs, digestive processes, and potential immune reactions so that when you do reintroduce an eliminated food and experience a reaction, you'll know just what caused it. Please note that while you may be intolerant or sensitive to a particular food, sensitivities cannot trigger anaphylactic shock. There is a difference between sensitivities, intolerances, and allergies (see Identifying Food Intolerances, Sensitivities, and Allergies).

The key to controlling inflammation is becoming aware of the problem and avoiding the causes. For Reset 90/10 to be effective, you will need to completely eliminate the following foods for three weeks. This protocol, while strict, is for healing, progress, and development, and I strongly encourage you to follow it as precisely as possible. You still have a 10 percent window that allows for slight modifications, mistakes, or situations where you might not have a choice. This is the beauty of the plan. Would it be most effective to be devoted to eliminating these items? Yes, of course, but life happens. You cannot possibly prepare for every situation, but try your best and remind yourself that you are doing this to change habits for the better.

Remember, you are what you *can* digest. If you cannot digest food properly, the same goes for anything else—pills, supplements, powders, or even gut-friendly kombucha may be fruitless attempts. If you have food sensitivities or too much harmful bacteria, almost anything you eat or drink could be perceived as an invader or cause discomfort. Invaders set off immune responses and keep your body out of balance. Until you calm your body and balance your microbiome, pills, detox kits, and short-term prepackaged cleanses (that are probably full of sugar alcohols, preservatives, and fillers) will never provide long-term results. With this Reset, progress looks like better sleep, balanced hormones, losing stubborn weight and bloat, less anxiety, clearer skin, improved digestion, and an adequately supported immune system. This jump start will help build a new foundation for better lifestyle practices.[18]

FOODS TO ELIMINATE

Alcohol is a toxin. When it enters the bloodstream, it impacts every organ and interrupts the body's normal processes. Alcohol also contributes to an acidic environment throughout your body, and the opposite of acidic—alkaline—is the key to essential health. Take twenty-one days off from alcohol and see how your body reacts.[19]

Animal meats are the hardest to digest and can cause inflammatory responses within the stomach lining. They are also a significant source of pathogens like salmonella, *E. coli*, listeria, and vibrio. It's clear that we need to reduce toxic chemicals in our food sources, and awareness of the issues is a start. But since the meat industry has a long way to go, I recommend consuming only organic, grass-fed meats for higher vitamin and antioxidant content. Grass-fed beef also contains significantly lower levels of saturated fat compared to grain-fed versions. These improvements come with a higher price tag, but the incentive in Reset is to introduce the benefits of more fiber into the diet. One could embrace this objective by balancing more vegetarian options into the weekly rotation and smaller portions of animal protein after the elimination phase.

Caffeine interrupts the normal function of insulin in our bodies. It also affects our adrenal glands and disrupts hormonal balances. When eliminating coffee, it is typical to experience headaches from withdrawal. This is normal and part of the detox process.[20]

Dairy equals inflammation, acidity, and hormonal imbalance. Digestive enzymes are created by the pancreas and are necessary for digestion. Lactose intolerance, a common issue, leads to malabsorption due to insufficient lactase enzymes, which could be caused by age, celiac disease, stress, medications, Crohn's, IBS, or diabetes.[21] Whatever the cause, without proper stomach acid and digestive enzymes, our body's ability to break down food is compromised, and we do not absorb nutrients. Undigested foods are often the beginning of many chronic health issues.

Eggs commonly cause food sensitivities. Your gut lining is thin and easily damaged. When the barrier of the GI tract becomes more permeable and is not in tip-top shape, the immune system fires up and food sensitivities occur. When food particles are absorbed into the bloodstream instead of the cells, this causes leakage and whole-body inflammation.[22] Eggs fall into the category of an immunoglobin-G (IgG) reactive food, as do wheat and dairy. An IgG immune response perceives foreign food proteins as adverse. When and if eggs are reintroduced after Reset, your chances of pinpointing potential sensitivities are considerably higher.

Some *fish* may contain more toxins than others, but during Reset, we eliminate them all. While there are many benefits associated with consuming fish, there are risks that come from contaminates from household and industrial wastes that end up in our rivers, lakes, streams, and oceans. Shellfish and bottom-dwelling fish can be highly acidic because they are more likely to have higher levels of pollutants. These adverse substances settle to the bottom where smaller fish and mollusks feed.[23] Pollutant examples include vehicles, chemical plants, your local mechanic, and construction sites. Larger fish tend to absorb more harmful chemical compounds because their food sources are the smaller fish. If mercury accumulates in your body, eating larger fish on a regular basis may contribute to your body holding on to this toxic metal. The good news is that mercury can naturally leave the bloodstream if avoided for six months to a year. After the Reset phase, reintroduce better quality choices, such as wild-caught instead of farm-raised salmon, which tends to harbor more pollutants. Also, avoid eating the skin and fat on fish, as contaminates concentrate in the fat of the fish. Again, reducing pollutants needs to start with a cleaner water supply. Educate yourself on how this can happen in your region. Knowledge is power.

Gluten and corn and soy are significant inflammation contributors, and their lack of quality suffers from blatant pesticide use. Recent studies have measured significant levels of glyphosate contamination in urine samples, which are associated with nonorganic food intake and adverse lifestyle choices.[24] Controversy and concern over this widely used pesticide suggests many detrimental effects on human health.[25] The negative impact of glyphosate used in these crops especially is linked to celiac disease, gut dysbiosis, malnutrition, and the suppression of vital digestive enzymes. Over time, this dysbiosis elevates with more serious comorbidities.[26]

Nuts and beans, while nutritious, are quite a task for the gut to handle in the healing stage. Cut them out for just three weeks to give your body a break and rest your digestive system. There are plenty of other plant-based protein options that we'll explore in the Reset phase.

Sugar is what I call the silent killer. Sugar causes more acidity in the body than it's worth. This means no sugar substitutes, sugar alcohols, or processed sugars. Raw honey and maple syrup are allowed in moderation as they provide nutrients and have antiviral, antibacterial, and antifungal properties.[27]

FOODS TO AVOID

While on my journey to better gut health, I was under the care of several different doctors and eliminating trigger foods was challenging because of the many conflicting protocols. Plus, I noticed that certain recommended animal products and fermented foods caused me even more distress, and I feared my relationship with meals was becoming disordered. Long-term management was my goal, and my research concluded that these different protocols had to be tweaked to support my needs, wants, and beliefs around food, without stress or eating meals that simply did not appeal to me. I decided to go back to basics. What was in the food I was eating anyway? I started to scrutinize labels and pick convenience foods with the least amount of ingredients. As the process unfolded, I learned that many of these everyday go-tos negatively alter the gut microbiome with inflammation.

So, in addition to the foods we just discussed, there are other ingredients known to cause an inflammatory response. Be mindful moving forward now and into Maintenance to avoid these as much as possible. Long-term use of many of these convenience items will negatively impact our gut microbiome.

Canned foods are often filled with MSG or other preservatives; canned soup is really just a big bowl of chronic inflammation. Make your own. I'll give you the recipes!

Most *condiments* are high fat with tons of sugar and salt, added dyes, fillers, and ingredients like high-fructose corn syrup, MSG, and soybean oils.

Convenience foods that use broad terms on their labels such as "natural flavorings," "carrageenan," "emulsifiers," or "binders." These generic terms can indicate almost anything, such as sugar alcohols, polysorbate 80, eggs, or dairy alternatives.

Dyes and preservatives are often unnecessary and cause significant damage to our gut lining.

Food allergens will mostly be eliminated in Reset. Down the road, if you suspect something you ingest is causing issues, I suggest restricting exposure entirely.

Fried foods are typically high in trans fats due to being cooked in oils at very high temperatures. The more fried foods you consume, the higher your inflammatory markers and the higher your risk of diseases like cancer, diabetes, and heart disease.

Omega-6 oils like corn, safflower, soy, canola, peanut, cottonseed, and grapeseed are best in moderation. While beneficial in small amounts, the overuse of these oils is highly inflammatory and promotes chronic illnesses. Read the labels of your favorite snack items, as these oils are often used in packaged foods.

Salad dressings with heavily processed and hydrogenated oils such as vegetable, canola, soybean, and corn. Other inflammatory ingredients would be listed as maltodextrin, monosodium glutamate, natural flavors, artificial flavors, and anything ending in "ose," which indicates a form of added sugar.

Packaged food items with butylated hydroxytoluene (BHT). This is an additive used to preserve food. Look for this ingredient in your chewing gum, snacks, cereals, dried meats, potato flakes, enriched rice products, and shortening. It is also commonly used in plastic and cosmetics—yuck! Long-term use has been linked to thyroid, kidney, lung, and blood coagulation disorders. This additive is also banned throughout Europe, Japan, Canada, and New Zealand.

Soda really has no benefit other than the fact that you like the sugary taste. You open the door to more acidic and inflammatory responses with every sip, so don't bother. It is not worth the risk.

White (refined) and processed grains such as bread, pasta, cookies, and crackers. Grains are made of three parts: the outer shell filled with fiber, vitamins, and minerals (bran); the carbohydrate layer (endosperm); and the core that's packed with unsaturated fats and vitamins (germ). Anything refined is stripped of the bran and germ—all the good stuff!—resulting in foods that break down very quickly. The faster the food breaks down, the faster our blood sugar levels rise. Next comes the spike in insulin, which, if in excess, leads to inflammation. Be sure to check the labels of your favorite packaged cereals and instant oatmeal. While they might say "whole grain" on the box, some of these products are made cheaply with corn, fillers, additives, highly processed sugars, BHT, artificial colors, and GMOs.

> For a product to be 100 percent whole grain, it must state that specifically on the package. For example, "100 percent whole-grain oats" or "100 percent whole wheat." Simply using the wording "whole grain" is another cunning attempt to lure the consumer in with less than average quality.

PRODUCTS AND OTHER THINGS TO AVOID

With the Reset protocol, I gave my body the break it desperately needed. I realized that less processed food equaled feeling better, so focusing on plant-based whole foods was the only way to go. From there, it was an easy step to recognizing other areas of my life where I could eliminate sources of inflammation. Remember, *removing* inflammatory response triggers supports *repair*. Look around your home and aim to keep these potential irritants to a minimum.

Chemicals in household cleaners (ammonia, ethylene glycol mono-butyl acetate, sodium hypochlorite), air fresheners (ethanol, formalde-hyde), and scented candles (benzene, toluene) could be messing with your endocrine system and causing hormonal imbalances. Disruptions happen because some chemicals mimic natural hormones and fool the body into overstimulating hormones like insulin when they're not needed. Pick fragrance-free options for cleaning products, garbage bags, and laundry detergents. For cleaning, you can dust surfaces with a damp cloth or use diluted white vinegar. You can help purify the air with houseplants or fresh flowers. To eliminate odors without conse-quences, use natural options like baking soda in the refrigerator, citrus peels in the garbage disposal, and a few drops of essential oils in a spray bottle filled with water.

Chemicals in personal care items such as formaldehyde (found in cosmetics), glyphosate (in weed killers), and oxybenzone (in sun-screens) are all known to be endocrine disruptors. Phthalates, a class of chemicals typically found in fragrances, will mess with hormones. Pick fragrance-free options whenever possible.

Medications—first things first: never stop a prescribed medica-tion without a doctor's consent. But be aware that long-term use of over-the-counter pain meds such as ibuprofen (Advil) and acid block-ers can cause significant damage to the permeability of the stomach lining. Continual reliance on acetaminophen (Tylenol) can be hard on the liver and can trigger stomach cramps and nausea. If these nonpre-scription meds are something you rely on out of habit, consider alter-natives like stress reduction, finding the root causes of inflammation with the help of a practitioner, or dietary changes to reduce symptoms.

Plastic containers unless they specifically state that they are BPA-free.

Stress and other emotional irritants are just part of life, and man-aging our responses is a work in progress. Your homework during the next several weeks is to become more in tune with self-care acts and to create a peaceful habitat. Preventive measures and a deeper consciousness of your surroundings support optimal functioning during this journey.

Tobacco causes increased inflammation throughout the body. It's no secret that using tobacco is bad for our health, yet we still support an industry that packages these extremely expensive, toxic, and addictive items. With over six hundred ingredients in a single cigarette, when burned, over seven thousand chemicals are released into the air. Breaking that habit comes with so many benefits, such as adding years to your life, improved breathing, more energy, and substantial financial savings.

CHAPTER 3

Replace

Let's now focus on all the better choices that promote healthier bodily functions! One of the most advantageous outcomes of Reset is eating more fruits and vegetables without fear, conflicting restrictions, or judgments. Though "elimination" might be a scary word, I promise you won't go hungry on this plan. Instead, nourishment and feeling satisfied have equal value. Think of the three-week elimination phase as a learning experience about what works best for you. We focus on feeling content, choosing easy-to-digest foods that won't cause insulin spikes, and keeping liver functions optimal so that cells can absorb the energy needed to keep your body working smoothly.[28]

Vegetables should take center stage in most meals. Focus on foods that are as close to their natural state as possible, as these are rich in nutrients and void of chemicals and additives. Plant-based, fiber-rich, and easily or slowly digested food choices are key.

The heavily processed convenience foods discussed in the previous chapter simply do not provide adequate nourishment. The food suggestions in this program offer optimal sources of energy and supply a range of nutrients. In addition, these foods contain prebiotic fiber, healthy fats, protein, minerals, complex vitamins, and antioxidants.[29] Perhaps you have heard that fruits and vegetables are high in carbs and sugar, but if we leave them out, we're neglecting the fiber, minerals, and vitamins they provide. One may think that fiber-rich plant-based carbohydrates are fattening, but gram for gram they contain half the calories of fat.[30] Even the US Department of Agriculture and Department of Health and Human Services agree; their Dietary Guidelines Advisory Committee states that plant-based, high-carb diets improve overall health.[31]

In addition, lower fat options aid in detoxing your body, optimizing liver functions, and getting energy into your cells. Reset foods will help you sleep better, knock out inflammation, eliminate cravings, and reestablish what healthy truly feels like for you.

Anyone can benefit from a plant-based shift, but remember that this is not an all-or-nothing mandate. If at the end of three weeks you have incorporated more plant-based options into your daily routine and want to keep it up, then mission accomplished!

AVOID FOR RESET (BUT ADD IN LATER!)

There are a few veggies you should avoid for the three weeks, though they do offer an array of health benefits and should be added back in for the Maintenance phase and beyond. No cruciferous vegetables (e.g., cauliflower, broccoli, brussels sprouts), please, as those are a little harder on your digestive tract. Anything that has skin (e.g., apple, sweet potato) should be peeled, as digesting skins is too hard a task in the healing stage.

If you have been diagnosed with IBS or SIBO, there might be certain fruits or vegetables on this plan you should consider staying away from as you Reset. For example, asparagus, butternut squash, and peas are often eliminated. Fruits like apples, mangos, and dried fruit will cause distress for some. Onions, garlic, and most vinegars can also be resistant to digestion. They may irritate your stomach or cause gas, bloating, and abdominal pain. For ideal results, most recipes in this book can be made without these ingredients until after Reset. Anything more than a half-cup serving of any irritating foods can cause distress to someone with a compromised intestinal tract.[32] I suggest experimenting here. The less irritation your gut experiences, the faster it can heal. If something bothers you, eliminate it.

GET TO KNOW CARBS BETTER

You're not alone when trying to figure out the many different forms of carbohydrates. There are three main types of carbs: starch, fiber, and unprocessed sugar. Try not focusing on what society, influencers, and our gym buddies tell us when it comes to the benefits or pitfalls of fruits and vegetables. In Reset, we attempt to sway that mindset and find what works best for us, as individuals, for optimal health.

With the Reset protocol, we ingest fiber-rich fruits and vegetables that provide instant energy for cells while still maintaining balanced blood sugar because of their fiber content. Complex carbs that exist in many of these recipes—including grains, vegetables, and fruits—are principal sources of energy. We are benefiting from the hydrating aspects of many of the fruits and vegetables we are ingesting daily, supporting a healthy digestive tract, and feeding beneficial bacteria with a balance of starchy vegetables. In addition, we benefit from polyphenols, antioxidants, vitamins, phytochemicals, and minerals, all while calming the GI tract to strengthen immune responses, the proper breakdown of nutrients, and our precious microbiome, hormones, and vital cognitive functions.

STARCH

Starchy foods play a significant role in our digestive health. The key function of these resistant starches is to pass undigested through your small intestine in order to ferment in the large intestine where they nourish good gut bacteria. This is a very important task!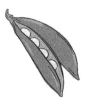

You will see that many of the recipes in this book include starchy veggies such as butternut squash, beets, green peas, sweet and white potatoes, and turnips to help stabilize bodily functions. Other featured foods include dried beans, lentils, and grains like oats and rice. In this journey, you will learn how more plant-based foods play a crucial role in the well-balanced, disease-fighting, and nutrient-rich options we can rely on as we Reset and build better, sustainable habits.

FIBER

Inadequate dietary fiber contributes to an imbalanced microbiome and complications in the colon, which can lead to short- and long-term illnesses. Without proper fiber intake, blood sugar fluctuates and opens the door to issues such as higher cholesterol levels, increased blood pressure, weight gain, and type 2 diabetes.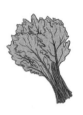

In our quest to balance and properly nourish our bodies, we need the complex structure of slow-digesting fiber to curb hunger and aid in limiting the desire for sweet treats on a regular basis. A diet that includes fiber-rich foods tends to mean fewer calories and more nutrients, which minimizes cravings and leads to healthy weight loss. Another benefit of fiber is short-chain fatty acid (SCFA) production. SCFA compounds are produced in the intestinal tract during the fermentation of insoluble fiber from plants.[33] More and more evidence reinforces the link between SCFAs and a healthy microbiome, proper liver functions, and blood sugar management. The health-promoting effects of these SCFAs include a reduced risk of diabetes, inflammatory diseases, and cardiovascular diseases.[34]

Soluble and Insoluble Fiber

SOLUBLE	INSOLUBLE
Dissolves in water and slows down digestion to give you that "full" feeling.	Adds bulk to diet and helps with constipation, has a laxative benefit.
OATMEAL LENTILS APPLES ORANGES	BARLEY COUSCOUS BROWN RICE
NUTS FLAXSEEDS BEANS DRIED PEAS	ZUCCHINI BROCCOLI CABBAGE
CUCUMBERS CELERY CARROTS	GREEN BEANS DARK LEAFY VEGETABLES ROOT VEGETABLE SKINS

Most plants contain both soluble and insoluble fiber. Both serve a purpose and are essential for healthy bowel movements, but do not overthink this. Your goal is to get more fiber into your diet. Too much processed or refined carbs, fat, or protein will bind us up. When stools are loose and watery, dietary fiber can help by solidifying the stool and keeping that colon clean. Soluble fiber dissolves in water, slows digestion, and forms a gel-like material, so when it passes through the colon, it feeds good gut bacteria as a natural prebiotic. This helps nutrient absorption and improves blood glucose and cholesterol regulation. Foods high in soluble fiber include avocados, berries, celery, dried fruits, legumes, rice, root vegetables, and whole grains.

Insoluble fiber attracts water to the stool and adds bulk, increasing the weight, size, and softness of your bowel movements and thus making them easier to pass. Insoluble fiber cannot be digested by bacteria but will stick to by-products of digestion, again making that function a pleasant one. Examples include apples, beans, barley, celery, carrots, citrus, oats, peas, and nuts.

Some over-the-counter bulk-forming laxatives have benefits, but most of these products are not advisable for long-term use. If you do not drink enough water with your stool softeners, more constipation could result. That promise of instant relief with packaged soluble fiber is a convenience that may give you more than you bargained for, with added sugar alcohols, natural flavors, and preservatives that, in the long term, cause much distress to the intestinal lining. Plant-based whole-food options, on the other hand, contain nutrients, hydration, and the essential fiber we need.

UNPROCESSED SUGAR

While I have made clear my feelings about processed sugar, natural sugars found in fruits and vegetables are a different matter. Unprocessed sugar found naturally in fruits are an excellent carbohy- 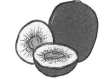 drate source as they are easily digested and can provide a healthier energy boost, especially first thing in the morning. That rapid release of energy comes from the food being quickly absorbed into the blood-stream, spiking an appropriate insulin release that then drops off as it should. If there is inflammation present, you may have to give your body, cells, and insulin responses time to adjust to the new routine.

CHAPTER 4

Reinoculate

What happens every day in our gut environment is extremely complicated. Research reveals new findings all the time, and what's clear today is that our GI tract performs a critical, complex task each time we eat, and that our intestinal health and its functions are vital to maintaining balance and overall well-being.[35]

Our gut microbiome contains a collection of living microorganisms (bacteria) called microbiota. Some bacteria are beneficial and essential for health and proper functioning throughout our bodies. Other forms of bacteria are destructive and don't belong in our gut habitat.[36]

Too many uninvited party crashers means trouble. Toxins, allergens, environmental factors, mold exposure, viruses, food poisoning, and an overabundance of unhealthy personal habits consequently drive what should be a well-orchestrated community out of control.[37] Without enough beneficial bacteria—and with too much harmful bacteria—we cannot break down foods in our stomach and metabolize vital nutrients. When there is less diversity of good bacteria and an increase of harmful bacteria, the environment is overly acidic and disease comes knocking. The Reset plan fights the harmful microbes and inflammation associated with certain foods by avoiding refined sugar, processed foods void of nutrients, additives, pesticides, and manufactured substitutes. Though these things make mealtime more convenient and quicker, they prevent the microbiota from doing their job efficiently.

Healing your gut is possible! And it's worth it because your gut environment has a profound influence on your overall health. It's important to remember that while plant-based food choices are key, this is also a time to prioritize better off-the-plate habits such as getting enough sleep and exercise and alleviating stress. Whole-body healing requires attention to self-care and preserving what is unique to each individual.

PREBIOTIC AND PROBIOTIC FOODS

Your food choices in this plan are full of prebiotic foods. Prebiotic-rich plant-based foods aid in nourishing and promoting the growth of beneficial probiotic microorganisms in the gut. Probiotics are living beneficial bacteria that naturally reside in the body.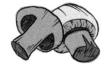

As we reinforce structure and calm, accomplishing the task of further improving gut health by introducing probiotics can be handled in two different ways. One is with quality probiotic supplements and the other is with the addition of nonpasteurized "live culture" foods like kombucha, kefir, kimchi, and sauerkraut. These foods or supplements are highly encouraged after the three-week Reset, but anyone, though especially those who are immunocompromised, should be mindful of fermented foods because of possible spoilage, mold, and fungal pathogens in what you make or buy. Know your sources, as the fermentation process is an art.

In addition, be mindful of when you add in probiotics, as you want to be sure your microbiome has a healthy balance. When introducing probiotic friends to unwanted bacteria, don't be surprised if a brawl breaks out. The good bacteria from fermentation is, at times, assertive in ridding the body of harmful bacteria. Common side effects of introducing fermented foods include gas, bloating, nausea, diarrhea, racing heart, and dizziness. Although the discomfort should be short lived, it will help if you slowly introduce probiotics in small increments.

ALKALINE VERSUS ACIDIC

If you are choosing empty-calorie, sugary, and high-fat foods on a regular basis, it may not entirely be your fault. That's because the typical standard American diet (SAD—how appropriate) is overly acidic. We consume more refined sugars and grains and half as many fruits and vegetables than are necessary for a healthy gut. When the body metabolizes foods made from processed flours, sugars, juices, and convenience items, it produces acid. Over time, an overly acidic environment creates an imbalance and the beginning of trouble for the whole body.[38]

TOO MUCH ACID

With an overabundance of acidic responses in the body, vital minerals like calcium, sodium, potassium, and magnesium can be taken from your bones to neutralize the acid and remove it from your body. When deficiencies are ignored and left untreated, symptoms can become more severe.

An overly acidic environment in your body is linked to yeast infections, acne, allergies, fatigue, and weight gain. When the issue is compromised further, more severe symptoms may include shortness of breath, ulcers, gastroesophageal reflux disease (GERD), nausea, immune suppression, low sodium, diabetes, obesity, kidney infections, osteoporosis, headaches, chronic pain, and confusion. It is also relevant to mention that the long-term use of acid blockers, while sometimes essential for relief, can cause a rebound effect when discontinued.

Bringing more attention to these facts is vital. The elimination of inflammatory foods and the introduction of more fruits and vegetables during Reset will aid in the process of bringing alkalinity back to optimal levels.[39] If we change the variables on the most crucial front, which is the overproduction of acidic responses and all the associated complications, the snowball effect of other ailments or need of meds and over-the-counter relief could be minimized considerably.

TOO LITTLE ACID

You now know that an overly acidic environment in the body is harmful. But so is the underproduction of hydrochloric acid (HCL), which is needed in the gut's habitat to begin the digestion process. The pH level in the stomach should be between 1 and 2, which is quite acidic because the cells that line our stomach secrete acid and release the vital enzymes responsible for the nutrient breakdown processes. In our stomach we protect our gut lining from self-digestion with a mucosal barrier. Maintaining this strong barrier with healthful choices is the goal. When we do not have proper HCL production, the stomach's ability to break down foods is compromised, especially the task of converting proteins into essential amino acids. The major role of HCL is to activate the secretion of a protein-digesting enzyme called pepsinogen (pepsin). These transformed amino acids are vital for functions throughout the body, so maintaining and understanding pH relevance is valuable information in this journey.

Stomach acid will naturally increase about twenty to thirty minutes into a meal. This process neutralizes enzymes from the mouth and kills any uninvited bacteria. That resilient stomach wall is also the first line of defense against harmful microbes and pathogens. Lower levels of HCL prevent the essential amino acids that plant- or animal-based proteins deliver from reaching our cells. Think of amino acids as physical therapy for our bodies. Without the proper conversion, we do not regenerate and rebuild. This creates chaos and can be the beginning of digestive health issues and infections.

Sometimes we inadvertently cause low levels of HCL. One common way this happens is when too much acid causes us to take over-the-counter acid blockers or prescription meds. When these are used in the long term, our vital stomach acid can become too low and the production of HCL becomes low or unstable. Once we go off these acid blockers, the rebound effect is for the body to overproduce acid. Subsequently, we need the acid blockers again and this vicious cycle continues.

BRING BALANCE BACK

The good news is that it is possible to create the healthy alkaline response needed to heal your gut, relieve your frustrating symptoms, and improve your well-being with gentle, knowledgeable guidance.

Acid Reflux: The Perfect Storm

Many of my clients come to me complaining about *acid reflux*, which can cause an uncomfortable burning feeling in your chest, neck, or throat and is often known as heartburn. Acid reflux happens when stomach contents move back up into your esophagus. Fun fact number one: if you have symptoms of acid reflux more than twice a week, you might have a condition known as gastroesophageal reflux disease (GERD). Fun fact number two: according to the National Institute of Diabetes and Digestive and Kidney Diseases, GERD affects one in five people in the United States. If left untreated, it can cause serious complications.[99]

Let's say you have acid reflux or a mild case of gastritis (stomach inflammation). Someone told you to stay away from spicy foods or citrus fruits. But you still have heartburn. Then you see a commercial that promises instant relief with an over-the-counter H2 blocker. You say, "Sign me up so I can grab the hot sauce and down that spicy margarita!"

You begin popping these H2 blockers like candy. They work immediately. Your doctor also prescribes a proton pump inhibitor (PPI) to stop that constant burning. A PPI works by blocking a system of cells in your stomach called the proton pump. In a nutshell, stomach acid becomes less acidic, more alkaline, and provides relief.

After five months, you run out of prescription meds only to discover that the reflux has come back with a vengeance. You thought you were cured. But actually, you've experienced a rebound effect from coming off the meds. Now you have more discomfort and more reflux. Your body tries to neutralize the acid on its own by leaching the minerals (calcium) from your bones, which puts you at risk for osteoporosis! Other potential adversities associated with long-term PPI use include deficiencies, kidney impairment, confusion, and the possible progression of dysplasia or tumor formation.[100]

At your six-month follow-up visit, your doctor concludes

that "this PPI is something you will probably have to stay on for the rest of your life." Fast forward five years, and you are complaining to your doctor about eczema, diarrhea, migraines, and bloating—all of which are symptoms of leaky gut syndrome.

Leaky gut, along with gastritis and ulcers, causes microscopic tears in the lining of the small intestine. Therefore, food particles go undigested into your bloodstream where they don't belong. Your immune system perceives these food particles as invaders and responds with antibodies. Over time the smaller holes can become larger and allow more harmful substances to enter your system, causing considerable damage to your health. And, with the overproduction of antibodies, the immune system grows tired and weak. Your doctor tells you that the stomach acid in your gut is now a pH level of 4 instead of between 1 and 2, and your protein, B12, zinc, and folate—which support immune health—are deficient.

With the overproduction of acid, your doctor tells you that this time, instead of mild gastritis (which could have been corrected with diet and lifestyle adjustments years ago), you have either a chronic illness like GERD or an ulcer. When left untreated, the snowball effect is malnutrition, a lack of serotonin, and adrenal fatigue. The cascade of symptoms opens the door to food intolerances, sensitivities, depression, and the onset of autoimmune illnesses. Give it another five years and it could even turn into the onset of esophageal or stomach cancer.

These scenarios don't have to have unhappy endings. Finding pH balance involves the conscious elimination of inflammatory foods and harmful situations. Incorporating alkalinizing food choices and practicing more supportive lifestyle activities reduce your stress load and decrease your exposure to toxins, resulting in balanced pH levels. No matter your gut situation, you can take numerous actions now to support whole-body health.

In Reset, with the elimination of inflammatory foods for a three-week period, we create a more alkaline environment for the body to thrive. When the body becomes more alkaline, we can also support the healthy acidic environment of the gut. First, we must address the overly acidic lifestyle choices that could potentially intensify any current gut issues. We can then establish if low HCL could be a potential problem that needs more attention (see Adequate Stomach Acid). Most often though, it is a combination of all the above, and starting with your very first drink every morning during Reset, you'll be working toward a more balanced and healthy gut.

You are on your way to significant improvements, better digestion, and the absorption of crucial minerals and vitamins through better food choices and lifestyle improvements. By significantly reducing or eliminating sugar and caffeine, your body will respond by maintaining vital blood sugar levels. It is equally important to not skip meals and drink plenty of water to support natural detoxification.

Remember, other factors that contribute to high acid responses in your body include stress, tobacco, alcohol, medications, excessive exercise, and lack of sleep. Billions of cells in your tissues rely on you to provide the alkaline environment needed to function correctly. Fortunately, improved nutrition and healthy behavior changes can jump-start whole-body wellness and support proper balance. Let's get to it!

CHAPTER 5

Repair

An integrative approach to wellness is about looking beyond the physical issues to facilitate whole-body healing. You are more than just a physical form, so a whole-body approach also incorporates mind, spirit, and community. Long-term sustainability, preventive action, and a balanced plate create a solid foundation to support this vision. Engaging with the physical, emotional, and nutritional sides of wellness is complimentary to the integrative medicine model.[40]

Balance goes so much deeper than what's on your plate. Food is essential, and you will learn about better food choices, but the core of a whole-body approach is a deeper understanding of what harmony means to you. How much time do you devote to exercise, your faith, meditation, being kind, joy, your social life, or self-care practices? Is your commute home from the office more stressful than a day at work? Are you clenching your jaw, feeling exhausted or emotionally drained, experiencing stomach or chest pains, or dealing with high blood pressure or headaches? Multitasking, chronic tension, and too much activity puts stress on our bodies and sends us into survival mode. This fight-or-flight mode affects the function of our thyroids, immune responses, metabolisms, and reproductive systems.[41] Awareness of your everyday stressors and how imbalances significantly affect digestion, hormones, and mood is good food for thought.

Please recognize that stress will also contribute to digestive issues and inflammation throughout your body. Think about what survival mode looks like for you. Are you barely getting through each day, exhausted and struggling to stay afloat? What changes can be made to get you off that life raft? Is asking for help difficult? Self-care is also a critical aspect of this plan. Cultivating a more peaceful environment where stress does not have you inhaling a sleeve of cookies is an aspect of what Reset can accomplish. When we calm our bodies with the best food choices and engage in self-care acts, we calm our minds. Is your mind at peace? Are you constantly on the go, not sleeping through the night, or perhaps excessively exercising, trying to rid your body of those extra pounds? At times, the body interprets excessive exercise as stress.[42] Exercise is essential, but anything excessive could backfire on those precious hormones.

Being constantly on the go with a never-ending to-do list that must be finished by the end of the day is no real way to live. In part 2 of this book, we'll focus on more self-care acts to balance life and make it more peaceful. Some days are easier than others, but you'll be invited to practice more skillful approaches to bridge physical and mental health. This could mean a daily walk, more meditative practices, the art of saying no, or resting more to recharge your battery. The goal is putting quality time into learning what works best for *you*. It's not selfish; it's self-care. That is a balanced plate.

Lasting change happens when you are all in. Not halfway in and halfway out or somewhere in between. Reset 90/10 jump-starts overall wellness by helping you let go of habits that may be harmful and then replace them with more positive, proactive, and conscious behaviors. It is not about perfection. Quite frankly, it's the opposite! It's about finding what works for you and letting go of the misinformation, trending diets, and whatever works for everyone else.

We are all looking for answers, better wellness, and happiness. We all struggle with something, whether it's trauma like death, divorce, or abuse; emotional issues like low self-esteem, obsessive behaviors, or depression; or physical problems like PMS, poor sleep patterns, or digestive issues. Even though you may not be able to shift your circumstances, the

So what exactly is too much exercising?

This question comes up often. There is a fine line between what is enough and what is too much, especially as age, health, and choice of workout must be factored in. A healthy lifestyle encompasses movement and daily activities for optimal heart health and overall mood.

The CDC recommends at least 150 minutes of moderate-intensity exercise and two days of muscle strengthening activity weekly for adults. If exercise exceeds three hours a day, causes distress, and interferes with other important activities, you may be overtraining and possibly preoccupied with that aspect of your life. Recovery can also be impaired by overexertion. Moderate exercise improves immune responses, while excessive exercise can suppress the immune system. If you are maintaining a regular schedule of reasonable daily activity, but are feeling anxious, blue, or out of control because you missed a workout, those symptoms are signs of withdrawal from what could be an exercise addiction.

Overexercising can also cause hormonal imbalances. At times, the body perceives excess exercise as stress. If someone has more than their fair share of stress already, their HPA-axis hormone production is activated. Overstimulation of the HPA is defined in more detail in this chapter, but basically, there is a call-to-arms reaction with negative hormonal surges. Despite your best efforts, this could mean weight gain, insomnia, night sweats, hot flashes, irregular or missed periods, dry skin, acne, unwanted hair growth, and irritability. Finding balance in how much you exercise matters, as too much of anything can come with serious consequences both physically and mentally.

good news is that you can make changes to alleviate some or all of the adverse symptoms. The desire to improve is what facilitates improvements. Action, consistency, support, and a positive mindset build lasting change.

One of the best ways to facilitate a goal is to write it down to give it true purpose. Another useful tool is the Circle of Life diagram (see the next section). Throughout this program you are invited to revisit your goals and spend time considering what you really want. In part 2, please see Try a Loving-Kindness Meditation. This is a positive daily affirmation that aids in overcoming self-sabotaging and negative thoughts or actions. An optimistic support system is highly encouraged because naysayers love to discourage. Consider writing yourself a letter of intent and keeping it somewhere you can view it daily as another motivational tool.

This book gives you the tools to succeed, but I can't be there to do your shopping, prep or execute your meals, make you exercise, schedule you a massage, or help you engage in mindful meditation. I offer education, encouragement, and tasty recipes, but action is up to you. Embracing that you are as unique as the next person will free you from a lifetime of misinformation and diets that don't work. You are your own best motivator, and motivation comes from within. Life will always present challenges, but if you approach them with positive thoughts instead of negative reactions, you will nurture your goals instead of discouraging them. What do you say we give it a try?

PRIMARY AND SECONDARY FOODS

Let's bring happiness back with better food choices, more calm moments, no regrets, letting go of the past, and a more precise outlook. With this mindset of foundational lifestyle improvements, the balance that is unique to all of us is possible. With that in mind, let's explore primary and secondary foods.

Primary foods are the things beyond the plate that bring joy and meaning to our lives. They refer to relationships, physical activities, spirituality, career fulfillment, emotional balance, pleasure, and love.[43] As stated, balance in our primary food category is unique to everyone.

When your primary foods are balanced and satiated, your life feeds you, making what you eat secondary (more on that in a little bit). To help you find your unique balance, please fill out the Circle of Life diagram. You can consider the following questions to get you started:

- Do any imbalances come as a surprise?
- How could you make time for any changes you would like to see?
- What help might you need from others?
- Which element needs the most attention?

Use this as a helpful guide to determine which aspects of your life you would like to improve upon. Aim for balance as you decide what to work on, and check in weekly as a gentle reminder to make positive change. Structuring balance should be a work in progress, as on any given day, one may find themselves hanging by a thread from life's uncertainties. As we become more balanced, we navigate those situations with a different perspective, leading to calm and clear responses.

At times, enlisting the help and perspective of a close, trusted friend or relative can help you balance your plate. Remember, friends who will love you despite your imperfections are the friends you keep close.

Another essential relationship is your healthy relationship with food. *Food fear* is a general fear of or anxiety about food brought on by media misinformation or conflicting views from family, friends, or acquaintances. The restrictions, guilt, shame, and obsessions that attach to a fear of certain foods can lead to compulsive behaviors or otherwise negatively control your life. Being in a toxic relationship with food can leave you feeling helpless and completely constrained. Restrictions with food will create havoc in your microbiome, dysregulate hunger hormones, and lead to nutritional imbalances. For example, I am constantly asked if eating a banana is okay. Many clients tell me they miss them terribly but are afraid from what they have read or heard on social media about trendy diets and reductionist theories that hold no credibility. The misconception is that this fruit should be limited in one's diet because of carbs, sugar, and calories. On the contrary, the evidence is clear that bananas are high in fiber, nutrients, and antioxidants and offer an array of benefits including digestive health, blood

Circle of Life

**Discover which primary foods you are missing and
how to infuse joy and satisfaction into your life.**

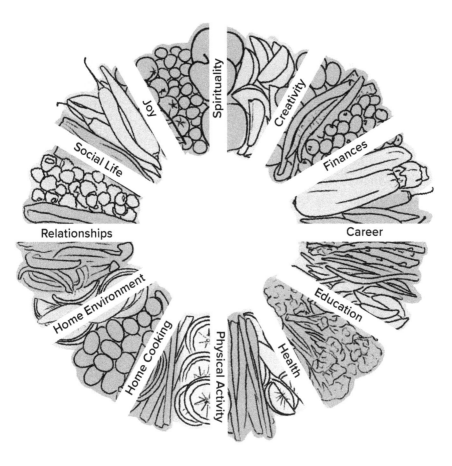

WHAT DOES YOUR LIFE LOOK LIKE?

1. Place a dot on the line in each category to
   indicate your level of satisfaction within each
   area. Place a dot at the center of the circle to
   indicate dissatisfaction, or on the periphery
   to indicate satisfaction. Most people fall
   somewhere in between (see example).

2. Connect the dots to see your Circle of Life.

3. Identify imbalances. Determine where to spend
   more time and energy to create balance.

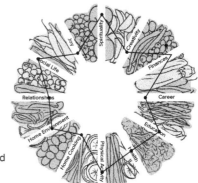

sugar balance, and heart health. Recognizing misinformation could mean cutting yourself off from views that don't align with your healthy values around food.

Secondary foods are the literal foods on our plates that hopefully nourish us. Food is essential, and Reset focuses on the importance of what, when, and how you eat. What is your state of mind at mealtime? Are you upset or calm? Can you genuinely say you thoroughly chewed your food and enjoyed the flavors? What about the planning and preparation of your meal?[44] Negative scenarios will unfavorably impact digestion.

If we put good intentions into feeding both primary and secondary foods, we have a better balance of supportive nutrition, hormonal health, and encouraging scenarios in every aspect of our lives. We satiate our hunger for food and life, and thrive knowing that nothing will ever be perfect and that's okay. Building a new foundation and circling back to these basics will benefit you thoroughly without the stigma of food fear.

THE GUT-BRAIN AXIS: CONNECTING FOOD AND MOOD

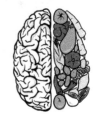

Broadly defined, the gut-brain axis is a complex system encompassing aspects of our enteric nervous system, immune health, the HPA axis, the parasympathetic and sympathetic nervous system, the vagus nerve, and gut microbiota.

Seventy to eighty percent of our immune health takes place in the gut. The protective barrier that is our immune tissue must stay resilient and protect the bloodstream from the external world. Too much bad bacteria will create an imbalance, but it goes beyond poor food choices. For example, if you are constantly worried or harboring unresolved issues, this stress will also control and drive that hostile imbalance in your gut. Comorbidities start and spiral out of control when there is no balance left.[45]

Your brain is also a vital force driving the health of your gut atmosphere. When our gut flora is imbalanced, the disturbance sets off a chain reaction throughout the nerves and up to the brain. It then affects our appetite, mental health, hormones, and regular elimination of toxins.[46] Without the proper intervention and mind shift that eliminates inflammation throughout the body, long-term consequences can include the onset of chronic illness and mental health disorders.[47]

Bringing much-needed attention to this rather complex system helps us understand how food options impact mood. Equally important are taking the proper steps to modify off-the-plate choices that can affect precious health.[48] When we are more aware of the gut-brain axis and its fundamental role in living a cleaner life, we can connect the dots and define our lifestyle goals. Change is possible; personalized nutrition is at the forefront of preventing and possibly treating disorders associated with diet, gut microbiome, and brain development.[49] Let's unpack a few relevant aspects of the gut-brain axis for a better understanding of what's going on inside our bodies.

THE VAGUS NERVE

The vagus nerve is the tenth cranial nerve, the most complex and longest nerve in your body. Referred to as the autonomic nervous system, it connects the brain, gut, intestines, and stomach. This nerve is a critical component of fight-or-flight mode and defines your entire body's hormonal harmony by controlling how quickly you can relax after stressful situations.

The vagus nerve is divided into the parasympathetic and sympathetic nervous systems. Our goal is to live more in a parasympathetic state of mind, as that is the system that supports optimal health, a calmer state of peacefulness, and the most robust digestive system.[50] While the sympathetic side plays an important role in increasing alertness, energy, blood pressure, heart rate, and breathing, these functions should only be utilized short term. Unfortunately, most of us consistently live with the sympathetic system turned on as we struggle with stressors 24/7.

Stimulating the vagus nerve can let your body know that it is time to relax. Regular practices like the ones that follow will strengthen your ability to shift from sympathetic to parasympathetic activity to allow for the rest-and-digest response. Long-term improvements can lead to less anxiety, greater overall well-being, optimal digestion, and supported immune system resilience.

- Deep and slow diaphragmatic breathing (see sidebar)
- Humming
- Singing
- Laughing
- Probiotics
- Meditation
- Exercise
- Cold compresses to the face and back of the neck
- Massage
- Connecting with nature

When your brain gets signals from the stomach via the vagus nerve that all is not well, it reacts negatively. Add stress, diabetes, anxiety, sugar, infections, unsafe cleanses, or improper food choices and the connection can be severed. Your brain stops getting the feel-good vibes from the gut, and these interruptions cause breaks in the permeability

The Vagus Nerve

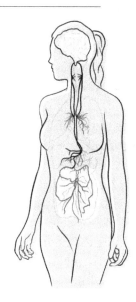

This superhighway of sensory nerve reactions needs support to properly transport robust functions from the gut, internal organs, and brain.

Recover from stressful situations with focus on a calmer gut environment, more harmony, hormonal balance, less inflammation, supported immune responses, and positive emotions.

Counterbalance the fight-or-flight reaction and stimulate the most favorable health benefits by assisting the body's response. Conscious rest and relaxation are necessary to strengthen this remarkable neurological function.

How Are You Breathing?

Did you know you should push your belly out when inhaling? Most of us breathe through our chest when, in fact, a *real* breath should come from our stomach. On the exhale, bring your belly in. This simple exercise practiced regularly supports the benefits of relaxation.

of your stomach lining. Potential symptoms of vagus nerve damage include difficulty speaking, chronic inflammation, heartburn, GERD, loss or change of voice, difficulty swallowing, low blood pressure, and a higher or slower heart rate.

When there is dysbiosis in your gut, you may not be absorbing nutrients optimally. Typically, blood markers will show increases and decreases, but they are not always a reliable predictor. If a client has gut issues, a drastic change in health, or prediabetic issues, I offer information on stimulating and supporting the vagus nerve. Please always communicate with your practitioners, but I also want to counsel the importance of self-care in every manner available. For me, the best possible outcome is a drug-free client who has exceeded all goals and sticks with a manageable, healthier lifestyle because they see it work and have never felt better.

For example, take IBS, SIBO, and other autoimmune diseases where gut issues are present. If your gut is off, the snowball effect is enormous and can negatively affect your thyroid, fertility, menopause, bone density, and nutrient absorption, to name a few. That said, it is essential to look at the symptoms and history of clients to inquire, for example, about typical bowel movements. We talk about it all, and it's surprisingly revealing. Proper elimination is also a significant part of healing.

By eliminating inflammatory foods and then slowly reintroducing them, you will find out quickly what makes you feel good and what doesn't. Stress also plays a massive part in determining the proper communication between the gut and the brain, the permeability of the gut lining, whether inflammation occurs, and the importance of the microbiome composition. In a nutshell, the connectivity is vital. Attention to improved gut health and day-to-day lifestyle practices nurtures your best physical and mental outcomes.

THE SECOND BRAIN

The enteric nervous system is typically referred to as the second brain. This considerable part of our nervous system occupies the walls of the long tube from our esophagus down to our anus and contains hundreds of millions of neurons responsible for controlling the gastrointestinal mechanisms within our bodies.[51] It converses with the brain in our heads and exclusively regulates digestive and absorptive functions. While there are many different communication highways in our bodies, keeping this specific avenue healthy is a critical aspect of well-being. Our resilient gut microbiome is fundamental to harmony and balance both cognitively and physically.[52]

Our gut microbiome contains stellar amounts of bacteria and microbes that live in the mucus lining of our intestinal walls. These microbes are in direct contact with nerve and immune cells, so chaos breaks out when there is too much harmful bacteria, stress, or a tear in that wall. In addition, 95 percent of serotonin is produced in the gut. When that "behavioral and mood hormone" is compromised, there is somewhat of a breach in security. The breakdown in communication from the stomach affects brain activity via the severed vagus nerve. A war breaks out within our bodies, and everything we consume is perceived as an invader. Powerful unattended inflammatory responses could lead to mood disorders like depression and anxiety, brain disease, hormonal imbalance, and gut disorders.[53]

THE HPA AXIS

Our brain controls cognitive behavior and chemistry. Our hormones (endocrine system) are responsible for regulating weight, aging, reproduction, and growth. When balanced, our gut (microbiome) controls our immune system. Without the balance, we risk autoimmune responses and inflammation. Understanding the impact of an unhealthy gut microbiome's influence on hormonal shifts and brain health begins with the hypothalamic-pituitary-adrenal axis (HPA axis), which regulates unified responses to stress.

The hypothalamus is a part of the brain that controls many bodily functions, including releasing hormones from the pituitary gland. The pea-sized pituitary gland is located at the base of the brain, close to the hypothalamus. The pituitary gland is a vital part of the endocrine system that produces hormones for various functions throughout the body.[54] The adrenal glands (which produce our primary stress hormones) regulate distress signals and control other necessary bodily functions, including metabolism and blood pressure.

An unimpaired pathway results in the proper production of cortisol. Genes, early-life development, and current bodily responses to stress determine cortisol activity. Rest assured, the release of cortisol in response to danger or stressful situations is beneficial. This natural fight-or-flight response is what has kept humans alert and alive in the face of danger. Unfortunately, when there is chronic stress, instability, and even the long-term effects of post-traumatic stress disorder (PTSD), the continuous pumping of cortisol can begin wearing the body down as it attempts to correct from within.

The parasympathetic nervous system facilitates an individual's repeated activation of this stress response either by curbing or allowing the unified reactions of the sympathetic nervous system and HPA axis. When the brain senses distress from the gut, the adrenal glands, being the primary hormone conductors, receive signals via chemical messages sent from the hypothalamus to the pituitary that there is trouble. Out pumps the cortisol and adrenaline, another hormone needed to keep you alert. Other organs and glands are affected, releasing hormones to help deal with the stress and return the body to homeostasis. Note how chronic stress compromises the following organs.

Pancreas (insulin): High anxiety activates the sympathetic hormones that elevate both cortisol and glucose. The continuous release of cortisol triggers the need for stored glucose from the liver to deliver fast energy during times of stress. Even if we haven't eaten, blood sugar levels are affected. Too much glucose in the blood turns into fat cells, which the liver stores, potentially leading to nonalcoholic fatty liver disease. High stress can also lead to insulin resistance. Glucose builds up in the blood because it cannot enter the body's cells normally—proper communication ensures that as glucose moves into cells, blood glucose goes down.[55] To compensate, the pancreas makes more insulin, and over time, blood sugar levels rise. A normally functioning pancreas makes more insulin when blood sugar is high and less when blood sugar is low.[56] Eating high-fiber, whole-grain, and low-fat meals helps slow digestion and take pressure off the pancreas.

Thyroid (metabolism): Constant fight-or-flight mode shifts the thyroid's function into a more inactive state, suppresses the digestive system, and affects insulin. This sensitive and cautious gland is the barometer of overall caloric adequacy in the body. The thyroid creates the hormones T4 and T3 to control metabolism, burn body fat, and distribute proper energy throughout the body.

Pineal (sleep): Being in a constant sympathetic state (always stressed or worried) will affect proper sleep cycles, compromising the body's ability to rest, repair, and grow.

Ovaries/testes (reproduction): A persistent state of perceived threat may affect fertility in a negative way. A disrupted connection between your brain and reproductive organs as a result of excess cortisol decreases blood flow to organs, which will affect ovulation and result in periods that are missed, irregular, or stopped altogether.

Thymus gland (immune): Chronically high levels of cortisol can affect this gland and thus the resiliency of our immune responses. Our ability to fight off foreign antigens is reduced, and we are more susceptible to infection and disease.

All these chemical responses cause symptoms such as weight gain, sadness, fatigue, hormone fluctuations, chronic illness, depression, anxiety, and irritability. In addition, our GI tract is extremely sensitive to the ill effects of an overabundance of cortisol. Unstable responses from the gut could be nausea, heartburn, constipation, diarrhea, and abdominal cramping.

Let's take a look at some common stressors that might be overstimulating the HPA axis. Everyday stressors include career, family, emotions, and politics.[57] These are personal, and some cannot be avoided. But you can support recovery from these stressors so that your body can bounce back quicker. Physical stressors are more complicated, as they can snowball negatively throughout the body. Quality sleep is essential, but a lack of it will impair immunity over time. Blood sugar imbalances cause chemical changes and open the door to blood pressure issues, hormonal issues, diabetes, diminished heart health, nerve damage, and weakened immune responses. In addition, you have to consider environmental risks such as pollution, toxic mold, food preservatives, and pesticides, to name a few.

The HPA axis should be a continuous circle of unity, so being aware of how it works is the first step to homeostasis.[58] A harmonious routine of self-care, a fiber-rich diet (fiber regulates insulin), and a balanced lifestyle help support efficient brain, hormonal, and gut function. Only *you* will deliver the best fuel for growth (both mental and physical), strength, support, and resilience.

FEEL-GOOD HORMONES

The four primary chemical neurotransmitters (hormones) in the brain that affect happiness are dopamine, oxytocin, serotonin, and endorphins. Healing and giving strength to these vital hormones is possible. However, without supportive measures, the dysregulation of these hormones is theorized to be connected to depression, addictive behaviors, obsessive-compulsive disorder (OCD), anxiety, disrupted sleep cycles, attention deficit hyperactivity disorder (ADHD), and bipolar disorder.

Dopamine is often referred to as the "happy" hormone and is part of your brain's reward center and many functions including memory, mood, and motivation. It can provide an intense feeling of pleasure and is boosted by unprocessed foods, omega-3-rich foods, fruits and vegetables, nuts and dark chocolate in moderation, less-saturated fats, probiotics, regular exercise (nothing excessive, as extreme exercise can negatively affect adrenal health), quality sleep, sex, laughing, and good conversations.[59]

Oxytocin is the love hormone that controls aspects of the reproductive system and is associated with empathy, trust, sex, and good relationships. Hugs, music, a puppy, massage, solid friendships, meditation, and good sex can help produce this hormone.[60]

Endorphins are "nature's pain killers"—your body's response to ease pain and bring about calm and happiness. Regular exercise will help the brain release this feel-good hormone, and foods like oranges, strawberries, grapes, nuts, seeds, and chocolate (within reason) are also encouraged.

Serotonin is a mood stabilizing hormone. Irritability, sadness, anger, not feeling like yourself, and chronic fatigue come with low serotonin levels.[61] Some doctors may prescribe antidepressants to boost serotonin in the body, and at times, this is the best option. There are more serotonin receptors in your gut than in your brain. We can also boost serotonin naturally with supportive foods to optimize the resilience of our stomach barrier. For example, foods with tryptophan and the right carbs promote amino acid absorption and boost serotonin.

SUPPORT OPTIMAL IMMUNE RESPONSES

In a time where ill health puts us at greater risk for disease, supporting your immune system is critical. Reset 90/10 will aid in optimizing immune and hormonal functions.

Our immune system is our first line of defense against inflammation in the body. Inflammation controls the disease, and that environment resides in our gut. Structured immune health requires eating the right food, but also the practice of self-care, gratitude, and mindfulness. As self-care practices unfold, better habits are established and old habits become a thing of the past. Consistency is vital to strengthen this new lifestyle.

One may grasp the concept of Reset 90/10 with clear conciseness and openness to change. Another may bounce around using up that 10 percent window whenever possible. Either way works. Old habits are hard to break. There is no shame in falling off track, if you get back on the path having learned a lesson. Not getting discouraged when you take a detour here and there keeps you motivated to stay on the road you've envisioned.

Research has shown that a fundamental shift to more plant-based options is a major predictor of a healthier gut microbiome. Remember short-chain fatty acids and how your body needs intact forms of fiber to nourish the good gut bacteria that produce SCFAs? Short-chain fatty acid compounds are in abundance in this plan. The water and fiber in fruits and vegetables support friendly gut bacteria, provide energy, and keep your colon happy. Eliminating processed foods and increasing your intake of plant-based dietary fibers is the jump start.

CHAPTER 6

Common Inquiries

IS THIS A DIET?

No, the Reset 90/10 elimination program is not a diet. It's a safe way to reduce inflammation and build a more balanced microbiome in your gut. Some may think this is a diet because it requires the restriction of certain foods, but the restriction is only over a short period of time. A diet may help you shave off a few pounds, but long-term maintenance seems to be a dead end for most. It all becomes too restrictive and frustrating with the counting, weighing, unappealing powders, and pills. Most likely the result is that you'll put the weight back on. Sound familiar?[62]

In a world of many dietary theories, one's head could pop off with all the information, advice, fads, and protocols being promoted at any given moment. Misconceptions about ideal weight, the influence of social media, and negative body image all promote an unhealthy relationship with food.

This program differs from dieting because it sees real food as medicine instead of the enemy. Once the elimination phase is complete and as the healing process escalates, you will be confident and able to make better choices. You will become more in tune with your body's unique responses and select foods that best meet your needs. That's not a diet, that's a plan to create sustainable habits that last a lifetime.

When we don't allow freedom and flexibility in any aspect of our lives, we open the door for bad habits to take over, which only ends up causing shame. Just remember, there is no perfect. Strive for 90 percent dedication and 10 percent downtime. What will unfold is balance, vital gut health, and awareness of the best possible physical and mental decisions for you. Embracing that you are unique will free you from a lifetime of misinformation and diets that don't work.

The goal here is becoming more mindful of what "healthy" means to you. The basic principles of removing inflammatory foods and adding more plant-based fiber-rich choices is not a diet plan. It's a lifestyle practice worth exploring.

WILL I BE HUNGRY?

I have mapped out a comprehensive plant-based protocol that includes meals, snacks, tips, and suggestions for optimal digestion. Along with optimal digestion comes absorbing more nutrients, thus having more energy. We focus more on ridding the body of inflammation and bringing about balance without wreaking havoc on hormones. By nourishing correctly, we reduce inflammation, stress, and anxiety.

Please keep in mind that your meals should leave you satisfied. If you're not satiated, you're most likely not getting enough fiber or not eating enough throughout the day. Starchy foods will help heal your gut and reduce inflammation. They will also feed good bacteria and keep you full for hours without cravings. The right choices aid in keeping insulin and blood sugar levels stable. Also, remember to hydrate to avoid constipation.

Most of all, listen to your body. If you want two bananas instead of one, go for it. Start enjoying all the different ways fruits and vegetables can satisfy. Filling up on the proper food choices comes with experience, so you have to dive in! Remember, there is no error if you wander by a tray of brownies at a social gathering and get derailed. Bad habits are hard to break, but when we fall and get back up, we learn. As you get more into the fundamentals of this plan, you will have fewer of those moments. You will start appreciating a treat that has no refined sugars, additives, or preservatives, and you will see the difference in how inflammatory foods affect your body as you purge the bad and replace them with better alternatives.

At the end of three weeks, you will be more aware of how plant-based foods can assist long-term wellness. When well prepared for hunger with suggested foods, you'll eat when hungry and stop when full. Reset has no calorie restrictions, but careful consideration of what, when, and how you eat will yield the best results. Eating to nourish and listening to your body when it signals you are full comes with practice, patience, and an open mind.

WILL I GET ENOUGH PROTEIN?

If you eat various plant-based whole foods (vegetables, legumes, 100 percent whole grains, and fruits), it is doubtful that you will be deficient in protein. Also, it may be interesting to know that the Centers for Disease Control and Prevention reports that most Americans exceed dietary protein guidelines without trying.[63]

Protein plays a vital role in thousands of biological processes, including giving cell walls their structure, transporting and storing essential nutrients, repairing tissues (such as bones, skin, hair, and muscles), and helping the body rid itself of toxins and waste. Protein is made up of amino acids. There are NEAAs (nonessential amino acids) and EAAs (essential amino acids). Our bodies can make nonessential amino acids on their own, but we must get the essential amino acids from food. The good news is that plant-based foods contain all the essential amino acids. Concentrations vary from one plant source to another, so diversity is important.[64] Equally crucial is that our digestive system breaks down the protein molecules. If there is dysbiosis going on, your stomach and small intestine cannot release essential amino acids from the foods you consume. Think of it: you are spending good money and time preparing food, but if you are not absorbing vital nutrients, malnutrition still occurs. It does not matter where you get your protein or how much you consume until you take a step back, give attention to the matter, and heal.

We cut out animal protein during the Reset phase because meat slows digestion and clogs up the bowels. Another concern is that harmful bacteria can grow more on protein-rich foods such as meat and dairy products.[65] In addition, research suggests that saturated fat, which is more abundant in animal protein, promotes inflammation.[66] I do not encourage long-term elimination of animal proteins, but this process calms your gut and its negative immune responses, pinpoints sensitivities, and introduces more plant-based options into your diet.

You will learn about better protein alternatives than meat and dairy, such as

- Buckwheat—Buckwheat and Roasted Vegetable Tabbouleh Salad, Cream of Buckwheat Blueberry Cereal, Cherry Tomato Pasta, Buckwheat Pancakes
- Ground flaxseed—Pumpkin Buckwheat Cereal Muffins
- Ground hempseed—Energy Fruit Smoothie
- Peas—Yuzu Pea Puree
- Nutritional yeast—Spaghetti Squash with Nondairy Cheese Sauce
- Quinoa—Buddha Bowls

Fruits and vegetables that are high in protein include: apricots, asparagus, avocado, bananas, blackberries, cantaloupe, fava beans, guava, kiwi, lima beans, mung beans, oranges, peaches, pears, potatoes, and raspberries. After the Reset phase, you will be ready to introduce more plant-based options like basil seeds, beans, broccoli, brussels sprouts, chia seeds, chickpeas, lentils, nuts, pistachios, tempeh, tofu, and wild rice. Plant proteins are abundant, powerful, and nourishing, and the stomach and the small intestine easily digest them. If we cannot break down that colossal steak due to a lack of digestive enzymes or hydrochloric acid, those essential amino acids vital for healthy blood, healing, muscle building, absorption, and nutrition can't do their job and we will just create more imbalances.[67]

When there is dysbiosis, undigested foods ferment and release into the bloodstream, causing harmful bacteria to grow and good bacteria to dwindle. When good bacteria are outnumbered, our immune system grows weak. The damaging invaders colonize, causing a variety of symptoms, including gas, migraines, candida, parasites, deficiencies, constipation, reflux, GERD, indigestion, dry skin, hair loss, and lack of energy.

The bottom line is that improving gut health is essential. Through the process of eliminating triggers, the gut becomes resilient and less permeable, so fewer toxins, bacteria, and chemicals cross the gut lining into the bloodstream. When the gut is intact, the healing begins. All the above is the recipe for less inflammation in the body and a more robust immune system.

HOW DO I FIND THE TIME?

That is a great question! Finding time for yourself is a self-care act worth exploring. Your health is invaluable and adopting a more proactive attitude in every aspect of your well-being should be on your priority list. This program shouldn't feel like a chore; instead see it as a stepping-stone to a better awareness of what "healthy" looks and feels like for you. When we value something, we give it attention. Being responsible for your health should alleviate any guilt associated with taking care of yourself.

Getting into a new rhythm with your personal positive goal should be your beacon of light from this point forward. You control your time, so finding space in your life to facilitate Reset's protocol is up to you. It's important to foster self-reliance, but it can also be helpful to have a sound support system to encourage a positive change.

Communicate with your family or roommates and, if possible, delegate activities that drain you so you can focus your energy on Reset for three weeks. Surround yourself with people who support your decision to be healthier. In the end, don't worry about the naysayers and trust your instincts. You bought this book for a reason.

Time management is an important part of this process too. Think about how you currently use your free time—do you really need to scroll through social media for an hour or watch five episodes of that TV show? Set aside time to get organized with the shopping lists and schedule your prep days ahead so you can get everything done without stress. Create game plans and menus with the suggestions and tips throughout the book.

Being brave enough to break unhealthy habits and lower your risk of debilitating illness and chronic disease is about taking charge to create lasting change. If you keep using the excuse "I don't have time," you will start to believe it. Make excellent health a vital part of life, and time will come to you.

WHAT IF I CAN'T DO IT?

If you are unsure about your commitment level, you may need to spend some time reflecting on your priorities. It sounds harsh, but quite honestly, if you truly feel as though you can't do it, this may not be the right time for you.

We are all swamped, and some times of life are more challenging than others. Many clients speak to me about obstacles and situations they feel might hinder their success. I want you to ask yourself, *What's holding me back?* Could getting up an hour earlier give you time to prep meals for the day? What about asking for help from your partner or a trusted friend? Are there internal negotiations going on inside your head as to why you cannot commit to your health? Is it that you can't, or that you don't want to?

Modifying your typical routine can potentially cause overwhelm because it's pushing you out of your comfort zone. You aren't alone. It takes effort to transform and grow. I stress to all my clients to keep life as simple as possible during the Reset phase. There will be days for simple, quick meals and days for more elaborate meals and preparation. This will all unfold as it should, and if you take on more than you can handle, learn from the situation and change accordingly. Don't give up.

In addition to keeping it simple, expect to give your body a break. Your body is working hard and may be sending you signals that you need to rest—don't ignore them! During the three-week Reset, please pay close attention to your body and give it a rest. That might mean sleeping in or no excessive workouts.

This program is about taking a break, healing, and building a solid foundation without the frustrations, shame, and guilt we conjure up every time we start a new diet. Don't forget to embrace your individuality, as what works for someone else won't necessarily work well for you. As you set this groundwork, remember change is a work in progress, and ultimately a solid foundation for better health, decisions, and habits.

Fear can be a formidable obstacle when our self-confidence wavers. If you are doubtful at the gate, just remember that *you* are the only thing holding you back. Give yourself the gift of a one-day-at-a-time mentality and choose to finish what you started. Believe you can do it, and you will.

WILL I BE HAPPIER?

Do you eat to live or live to eat? It doesn't matter much either way. Would either answer guarantee eternal bliss? Doubtful.

The fact is that there are hundreds and hundreds of dietary theories out there waiting for you. Most of these fads are just money-making schemes that rely on you falling for gimmicks, pills, myths, and nonobjective studies. In a world of Google searches, gurus, experts, MDs, and YouTubers, will the answer ever be clear? It might not be.

So can you be happier if you follow the theories outlined in this book? I hope so. But the real question is, Are you satisfied now? Do you look in the mirror and like what you see, or do you want to look like that blogger you follow because she seems to have it all figured out? Guess what? She positively does not have it all figured out. As you Reset, pay attention to what makes you happy. What are your goals for the future? For myself, I want to be happy, full of energy, and the firecracker of health at age ninety. Also, always check in with emotional responses and stressors that may cause you to reach for salty or sugary comfort foods. Instead, go for a walk, call a friend, or find a distraction that brings you joy.

Embrace that being on top of your health is the most considerate thing you can do for yourself. Considering the pros and cons of any step I took toward better health and educating myself made this path perfectly clear to me. After making considerable strides in my health, putting more time into aligning my overall spirit and being grateful for what's right in front of me just clicked. Eliminating stress is a great goal, but as stress is all around us at any given moment, it's not what you get but more of how you handle it.

Here's something interesting to ponder relating to stress: we need the fight-or-flight response when something potentially threatening arises, as it improves overall alertness, performance, and memory. Good stress motivates us on a daily basis as every day is a new challenge with tasks, goals, and focus. Good stress is that feeling when your pulse quickens and hormones surge but there is no alarming threat. Connect that motivating feeling with the desire to improve your health. Your health is a serious issue, but nothing will ever be perfect, so if you can allow yourself that wiggle room right out of the gate, it's more likely negative stress and anxiety will decrease.

Even with modifications to food choices and a new outlook on and off the plate, I cannot guarantee your contentment. You hold the key to that, my friend! When you accept responsibility for your actions and make more deliberate choices, you can navigate life with a more concise mindset. Self-care goes beyond food, water, and exercise. Find your balance and the powerful healing associated with taking charge of yourself. That will be your stepping-stone to happiness.

PART TWO

The Reset 90/10 Program

Welcome to part 2 of *Gut Driven*! Now that you've become more familiar with how digestion works and the science behind the gut-brain connection, it's time to start the program. Part 2 is divided into four chapters that you'll want to follow chronologically:

Preparation. Do *not* skip this part. Properly preparing for the next three weeks is vital. In this chapter, you'll get prepared physically and emotionally for the program. You'll be asked to set goals and designate a support system. You'll also get tips for preparing your kitchen, ideas for menu planning, and a shopping list.

Week One: The Detox Stage. This is a vital step to rid the body of inflammation. In this stage, you will eliminate potential irritants, addictive substances, and processed ingredients. Detox is necessary to cleanse and break habits.

Week Two: The Honeymoon Stage. You'll experience the glorious feeling of settling into your new routine. You'll become accustomed to the new changes and hopefully more optimistic that transformation is possible.

Week Three: The Transformation Stage. In this stage you are more proactive, supporting this new attitude you have created. Old unhealthy habits may no longer interest you, and you'll favor those better practices. The opportunity for growth is in your path, and you'll welcome how in sync you have become with change.

In Reset chapters 8, 9, and 10, supportive components of your development will be built upon balance, awareness, and education. This framework repeats in each chapter under the headings "Get Balanced," "Be Aware," and "Stay Educated." Together, these action items set the groundwork for optimal well-being.

CHAPTER 7

Preparation

They say old habits are hard to break, but in three weeks' time, with dedication, you'll look back proudly at your accomplishments. This chapter is carefully laid out to set you up for success. When we create harmony where it was once lacking, we look forward, eagerly awaiting the road ahead. Reset 90/10 welcomes you to start this new journey hungry for change. This adventure of discovery is focused on your growth and overall wellness. Remember, you are capable of profound and powerful modifications with the understanding that you may have to stir things up, let stuff go, and settle in to allow for progress. It's like that wonderful feeling of cleaning out your closet. Let's jump in!

The Reset 90/10 program contains a complete meal plan for the next three weeks. You'll find food suggestions for breakfast, lunch, dinner, and snacks, along with a blank sample menu to use when planning your meals for the week.

My biggest wish is that you will have fun exploring all the delicious food combinations that Reset 90/10 offers as you decide on recipes and meal plans. However, I know the feeling of being overwhelmed by something that's out of your routine. That's why I've provided menu suggestions for each week of Reset. These are just suggestions. I encourage you to use the blank menu to plan out whatever works best for you!

You will find a comprehensive shopping list and a weekend prep planner. The two work together to help you be your most efficient. In case you are curious about food sensitivities, you'll also find an invaluable symptoms and food tracker chart in the back of the book, where you can keep track of your progress and any potential reactions to food. Planning, efficiency, and strategy are critical for any successful endeavor.

When you decide upon an official start date—whether that be tomorrow, the week after, or three weeks from now—consider making small changes and modifying your choices before your official start date to make the transition flawless or more efficient. For example, because of scheduling conflicts, you may choose to start two weeks from now. But that doesn't mean you can't get a head start! As you get familiar with new menus and protocols, consider modifying your habits or initiating the routine of drinking celery juice first thing in the morning. Or just start adding more fruits and vegetables to your rotation. Try not to get overwhelmed. Remember, true progress is made with small, consistent steps toward your goal. A common pitfall is wanting too much too soon, so let this plan unfold as it should. Let's get started with an overview of what the next three weeks will look like.

THE RESET 90/10 OUTLINE

STARTING YOUR DAY

Upon waking, brush your teeth. Quite a lot of bacteria grows in your mouth, especially while you're asleep for many hours, and you don't want to drink those harmful bacteria back into your body.

Each day, you will start with sixteen ounces of celery juice on an empty stomach. A juicer is best for this and other juice recipes, but you can also use a high-powered blender (see Celery Juice). Celery juice has received much attention as a super-elixir in the last several years for good reason. This alkaline juice will calm an acidic environment, jumpstart the detox process, support your hormones, and nourish with several impressive health-promoting phytochemicals.[68] If you have ever had strep, prescription meds for longer than two months, invasive surgeries, food poisoning, compromised periods, gastritis symptoms, or trauma, you may need the benefits that celery can provide.[69] Plus, celery juice provides hydration void of any adverse side effects. Drink up!

If you try the celery juice and do not like the taste of it, substituting cucumber juice is acceptable. In most instances, celery juice will grow on you, so I encourage you to give it a try for a week or so. Remember anything drastically different from your normal routine may take time getting used to. If you think that buying celery juice powder will get you out of juicing celery, I only wish it were that easy. As you focus on the hydrating benefits of fresh fruits and vegetables, it's essential to know these gimmicky, heavily processed, and cleverly marketed powders are void of the many nutrients fresh celery juice provides. Stick to the real stuff.

Your second ritual of the day is drinking eight ounces of warm water with a teaspoon of fresh lemon juice (Warm Lemon Water) about twenty to thirty minutes after the celery juice. Starting your day in this manner is a great way to wake up the body and alkalize further. Lemons (or limes if you run out) support and strengthen the immune system, help control high blood pressure, and regulate body temperature. If you feel constipated or nauseated, lemon water is also beneficial for the digestive tract. It is also ideal before and after a workout, as its benefits extend to the cardiovascular and muscular systems.

For optimal hydration, aim for at least sixty ounces of water a day. Always drink your water before meals, not during, as it disrupts digestion. If you want to add flavor, add a splash of lemon juice or fresh herbs (basil, thyme, mint, and rosemary are delightful). With this daily intake of water for three weeks, you will be doing wonders for your digestive tract, skin, mood, and kidney functions. Keep in mind that seltzers do not count as water, especially if additives or sodium are listed on the label. If you are experiencing any type of reflux, seltzer is definitely not for you.

Wait another twenty to thirty minutes before having your daily Energy Fruit Smoothie. There are no fats, MCT oil, or superfood mixes in this smoothie. Wait till after the Reset phase to start adding things like superfood powders. Fresh herbs are always encouraged as add-ins and aid in the detoxification process. If adding protein powder to your morning smoothie, please see the recommended brands in Pantry Nice-to-Haves. When considering other brands, please read the labels and avoid products containing whey (dairy), added sugars, sugar alcohols, fillers, and citric acid. There are many cheaply made products out there not worth your money. If you're looking for more protein during Reset, add a serving of ground hempseed to your morning smoothie. Hemp protein contains all nine essential amino acids and its protein composition is similar to an egg white but with the benefits of more fiber, calcium, iron, and healthy fats.

You'll learn more about this daily process in Benefits of Your New Morning Rituals in chapter 8.

MIDMORNING SNACK

Snack on fresh fruit if you are hungry sometime between your morning smoothie and lunch. For example, if you have your shake around 8:00 to 9:00 a.m., you might want to snack on a pint of blueberries around 11:00 a.m. or noon. Or try eating a whole mango or half a papaya. Sometimes I snack on a little of both, and that's okay. Try out an apple (peel the skin for Reset), an orange, or a banana. Watermelon is super hydrating! Cantaloupe, honeydew melons, dragon fruit! Grapes (peeling not necessary)! Try whatever is in season and available to you.

Fresh fruit should be eaten only as a morning snack. Fresh fruit on top of a cooked meal is an irritating task for the digestive system to handle appropriately. Food negatively ferments in our guts this way and causes many digestive issues.

Eating when you think you are hungry should not be a knee-jerk response. Pay attention to more intuitive cues, like stomach grumbling. Most of us mistake thirst for hunger, so with that in mind, ask yourself if you are drinking enough water before looking for a snack or another meal.

Remember to rest and digest as you enjoy the energizing benefits that fruit offers. The fiber in the fruit will keep your insulin levels from rising drastically, and you will feel energized with stable responses.

LUNCH

Please, please, please remember this important point: keep it simple. I cannot stress enough that for the next three weeks, you are restructuring your relationships on and off the plate, and it takes a lot of time

Top 10 Hydrating Foods

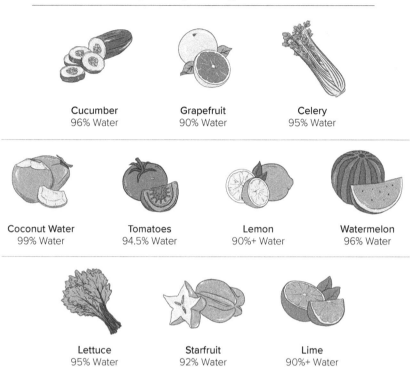

Cucumber	Grapefruit	Celery
96% Water	90% Water	95% Water

Coconut Water	Tomatoes	Lemon	Watermelon
99% Water	94.5% Water	90%+ Water	96% Water

Lettuce	Starfruit	Lime
95% Water	92% Water	90%+ Water

and focused energy. Your body will crave simplicity during this time of removal, replacing, reinoculation, and repairing. So do your body and mind a favor and give yourself a break—you are not auditioning for an episode of *Chopped*! Stress in the kitchen equals stress in the body.

Your lunch and dinner options will be similar. For lunch you might serve yourself Simply Mashed with a side of steamed asparagus and olives, which are all good gut foods. The Buckwheat and Roasted Vegetable Tabbouleh Salad is refreshing, purifying for the body, and filling. This salad will also hold up well in the refrigerator for days.

Soups are highly functional and a healthy way to fill up on veggies. Take your pick from the seven soup recipes in the Reset section. Soup can be lunch and dinner for several days, plus you can freeze leftovers. Try adding small amounts of white rice, whole-grain buckwheat, or quinoa to make it a heartier dinner option when you need a little more comforting nourishment. I've also included some breakfast-for-lunch-or-dinner options as an occasional choice.

AFTERNOON SNACKS AND DESSERTS

Dried fruits are perfect as an afternoon snack after cooked foods, in moderation. Try goji berries, dates, figs, mango slices, mulberries, and apricots. You will know quickly what you can or cannot tolerate. Gas is natural, but eliminate any dried fruit if you are incredibly gassy after eating it.

Besides dried fruit, try Pumpkin Buckwheat Cereal Muffins or Quick Applesauce (an unsweetened store-bought version also works). Make a parfait with applesauce and dried mulberries on top. It's delicious and doesn't require much planning! If you are worried about consuming applesauce after a cooked meal, know that cooked apples are easy on the digestive tract as opposed to a whole uncooked apple, which requires much more work to break down.

When you are thinking a snack or dessert sounds good, identify what kind of snack you are in the mood for. Many of us have a habit of reaching for sugary snacks quickly after a meal. If you are one of those people, try a date with tahini (Dates and Tahini). It's a delicious and satisfying way to kick that sugar habit to the curb. If you are missing your nightly bowl of ice cream, try the Frozen Banana Cream occasionally. It is truly scrumptious, filling, and will help you sleep with a healthy dose of tryptophan. After three weeks, you will not crave those sugary treats as much and will have more creative and healthier ways to indulge on occasion. A salty craving may be satisfied with a seaweed snack (see Baked Seaweed Snacks) or a rice cake with salsa.

After a delicious, filling dinner, don't rush to grab a dessert or snack right away. Give your body a chance to digest properly. If you are settling in for a good movie and want to nosh on something, Oven-Dried Mulberries would be my pick. It hits the crunchy and sweet notes for sure. As always, snack in moderation and give your stomach time to catch up to your brain.

DINNER

Healthy fats are a crucial part of optimal health, but for the next three weeks, we are aiming for low-fat, high-fiber, and starchy plant-based carbohydrates. Fat is reserved for later in the day after our liver cools off and can process the fat effectively. When our liver is sluggish and overworked, simple processes like creating energy, removing harmful toxins, making new blood, and utilizing nutrients are compromised. Healthy oils, coconut milk, avocado, tahini sauces and dressings, and olives are all excellent sources of fat in moderation.

Concentrate on easily digested meals and complex carbs to curb cravings, keep you full, and eliminate inflammation. Something like a pot of Ginger Pumpkin Soup is a well-rounded meal and not too difficult for chefs at any level. Another simple dinner suggestion would be to try roasted sweet potatoes or Baked Potatoes with avocado slices. Add to that a Simple Salad. These simple greens are crucial and what your body needs for proper waste elimination.[70]

Finally, you can also juice about an hour before bed. Celery and cucumber juices will calm the digestive system after a long day—the naturally occurring mineral salts in these vegetables aid in reducing acidity in addition to hydrating your body.

PREP FOR SUCCESS

Finding balance means developing a new understanding of what works for you specifically. It involves trying new things and taking action. This program requires effort, and you will be asked to get out of your comfort zone while testing different foods and incorporating new habits. That uncomfortable feeling associated with change is growth, so don't shy away from it! Let's prepare for success with a back-to-basics approach to the kitchen, meal planning, and goal setting. This is your chance to hit the reset button. Your goals are attainable, and mindfulness unfolds as you start taking better care of yourself—not just for three weeks but from here on out.

Time management is a key component of preparation. You choose how to manage what's important on your to-do list, and with Reset, cooking (and preparing to cook!) will need to be a priority. Even as you manage yourself more efficiently, you will realize that some days, getting everything done just isn't going to happen, and that's okay. If you're feeling overwhelmed, take a step back and see if there's anything you can take off your plate. You only have so much to give, and some days it will be less than others. There's always tomorrow to get back to it. Let's balance it all out and relieve some pressure on that never-ending agenda, shall we?

GET YOUR KITCHEN READY

You probably know by now that this plan will have you spending more time in the kitchen. Before you get cooking, set yourself up for success with a thorough cleaning so you can assess what you have, organize, and restock staples as needed. Creating a kitchen that's ready for success will give you a safe space to take on this journey.

Temptation is a constant struggle. If snacks or any other foods that will make you weak in the knees are present, get them out of your kitchen. Go through your pantry and any other hiding spaces and get rid of these foods to reduce the stress of unwanted invitations to crack. Enlist support from your family members or have them hide their addictions elsewhere for the duration. Remember, the more junk food you eat, the more you crave it. It's a vicious cycle, but it's one you are about to break.

When revitalizing your pantry, consider when you last bought dried herbs. It might be time for new ones; they lose their punch after a year. Another good test is to just smell them; toss if you don't get an aroma right away. If the elimination of coffee is already stressing you out, consider picking up some soothing, calming decaf teas such as mint, chamomile, lavender, lemon balm, and rose. Lemon-ginger tea is suitable for a pick-me-up and cinnamon tea helps cut sugar cravings. To aid in the digestive process, try peppermint, fennel, ginger-dandelion, and marshmallow root teas. Hibiscus tea is a tart, fruity tea that tastes similar to cranberries. Pomegranate tea is full of antioxidants and blood orange is pure refreshing citrus flavor. Keep in mind that decaf coffee cannot substitute for coffee. Decaf coffee beans go through quite a process to eliminate the caffeine, so let's skip it altogether during Reset.

Next, take a good look inside your refrigerator. Keep in mind that commercially prepared condiments, certain types of vinegar, and salad dressings have a lot of inflammatory oils, processed sugars, yeast, additives, and preservatives. Read all the labels and toss anything with these ingredients. Homemade is so much better, and I'll give you the tools to make them. Clean out the produce drawers so they are ready for new, fresh goodies. Having the fridge well organized and alluring will contribute to a confident, well-executed adventure. You might as well tackle the freezer while you're at it. Make it a point to clean out the refrigerator once a week and get creative with what's left. Those items in the back of a drawer can become an impromptu soup (see Hearty Vegetable Soup), stew, stir-fry, or savory roasted vegetables that you can have as a side dish or transform into vegetarian lasagna.

There are a couple of kitchen appliances that I highly recommend investing in if you don't already have them. If price is an issue, check thrift stores or other secondhand shops. I have found close-to-new juicers and blenders at these stores. Or ask your friends and family—someone may be willing to give you an appliance they never use. Even an inquiry on a social media site can save some money. Keep these gadgets on the counter or readily available as you will be giving them a workout from now on.

Rice cooker: Some rice cookers serve double duty and come with steamer attachments (see Steamed Vegetables) for your convenience, starting at around $30. There are also models that function as slow cookers and have the capacity to cook larger quantities of foods; these are pricier at $100 and up. I personally love my small, inexpensive rice cooker and use it to steam vegetables several times a week. Cooking grains is also a big time-saver and the results are mostly flawless. For me, this is a worthwhile and highly functional purchase.

Juicer: Store-bought juices are loaded with sugar, preservatives, and additives. These juices are most likely pasteurized and void of nutrients. Instead, investing in a good juicer is your best bet. Breville offers three types of models ranging between $130 and $380. I have found the higher-end version perfect for my needs. I juice celery, cucumber, and a combination of fruits and vegetables twice a week. During Reset, you will be juicing every day or every other day. If you think you will only ever use a juicer to make celery juice, then the least expensive model would be sufficient.

Blender: If a juicer is just not an option, use a high-powered blender. I have found that you don't have to break the bank to get an efficient blender system that can tackle many functions. My top pick is the seventy-two-ounce Ninja Mega Kitchen System. There are many pros associated with this affordable model, and making juice is one of them. For obvious reasons, the more power, the better, and this specific model gets the job done with some added benefits. The system includes two single-serve cups so you can make individual smoothies super efficiently. With the extra cup, prepping for your morning Energy Fruit Smoothie is simple. You can also use the individual cups to make salad dressings, pestos, and sauces. Other perks are its seventy-two-ounce capacity, the processor attachment that can rice vegetables, and a dough hook. To make your fresh juices in a blender, you will also

EQUIPMENT CHECKLIST

- ☐ Blender
- ☐ Cooking twine
- ☐ Cutting boards
- ☐ Mason jars with lids
- ☐ Immersion blender
- ☐ Juicer
- ☐ Mixing bowls
- ☐ Muffin pan
- ☐ Parchment paper
- ☐ Pots, pans, and sheet pans
- ☐ Rice cooker

- ☐ Sharp knives
- ☐ Spiralizer
- ☐ Storage bags
- ☐ Steamer basket
- ☐ Storage containers— see Souper Cubes in Resources for convenient and freezer-safe containers
- ☐ Sushi mat
- ☐ Vegetable peeler

PANTRY CHECKLIST

- ☐ Stainless steel, glass, or BPA-free plastic water bottle
- ☐ Apple cider vinegar
- ☐ Dried herbs and seasonings
- ☐ Coconut aminos

- ☐ Coconut vinegar
- ☐ Maple syrup
- ☐ Olive oil (good quality)
- ☐ Pump cooking sprays (avocado, coconut, and olive oil)

need a nut milk bag or cheesecloth (available online and in specialty stores) and a large bowl to properly strain the juice.

Spiralizer: Most home cooks love this inexpensive tool. You don't have to spend a lot on a fancy, costly machine; many online sellers have popular brands that retail between $30 and $40. Spiralizers not only turn fresh vegetables into faux noodles, but they also cut prep time down considerably by thinly slicing veggies into all sorts of different shapes and sizes. It's a time-saving investment worth looking into.

PLAN YOUR MEALS

Planning your meals is highly encouraged for several reasons. You have set a goal, and for the best chance of reaching that goal, you need to spend some time preparing. Meal planning ensures that you eat a variety of fruits and vegetables and meet your nutrient needs. Save your old planning menus throughout this process and compare your weekly food options for more diversity. It's interesting how we seem to settle in with the same meals week after week. Diversity with foods offers nutritional perks and the chance to find something new that you love, and reduces the risk of chronic lifestyle diseases.

With planning, you are more likely to reach your goals, save money, and control food waste. Efficiently outlining a meal plan could also save you time. For example, if you get ingredients to make a big batch of something freezable like soup, muffins, or buckwheat pancakes, future meals can be prepared in little to no time. I am a big fan of this kind of batch cooking, which is why some of the recipes yield larger amounts. You can also freeze freshly made juices. Consider purchasing freezable mason jars. You can defrost a single serving of juice overnight and save time in the morning.

Getting into the habit of meal decisiveness also prevents the frustration that typically leads to calling in for pizza delivery. As a chef, planning was a crucial part of my strategy, and it alleviated unnecessary stress while supporting skillful productivity and product utilization. Win, win, win! Consider what appeals to you, what is manageable, and what is realistic. For example, keep things simple by planning several meals with common ingredients. It is also nice to count on leftovers for helpful next-day options.

To help with planning, I've included three sample menus with ideas and suggestions for the three-week Reset phase. Also included is a blank menu planner to help with planning your meals. Find these at the end of this book; you can also download additional copies of the menu planner at www.chefellen.com in the recipe section. Fill out this handy planner, check pantry inventory, and adjust as needed prior to shopping.

PANTRY SUBSTITUTIONS

Even with a planner, please remember to be flexible! Items may not be in season or available, and if the lack of required ingredients for a recipe makes your head spin, don't sweat it. Make it a challenge. Trust what you learn in this book to guide you in selecting a substitute that'll be comparable. Keep in mind, as you become savvy in the kitchen, your confidence will grow when considering substitutions. When you think of a recipe component for what it is, substitutions can be easy (for an example of how to get creative when you're out of an ingredient, see Pumpkin Buckwheat Cereal Muffins). Instead of giving up, think in general terms of a swap, and taste as you go. Acids swap for acids. Sweets for sweets. Fire for fire. Texture for texture. The results of substituting ingredients can be magical, and they make the recipe your own.

- Vinegar? Use lemon or lime instead.
- Capers? Try olives cut into small pieces.
- Heavy cream? Try canned coconut milk. It's healthier and more easily digested.
- Mayo? Try a mashed creamy avocado instead and avoid all the preservatives.
- Oil for a muffin or quick breads? Try applesauce in the same 1:1 ratio.
- Peanut butter? Try tahini and support your thyroid.
- Buttermilk in pancakes? Use oat milk and a tablespoon of lemon juice to create the same flavor profile and texture.
- Raisins? Reach for cranberries or cut-up dates.

In-Season Produce

Spring	Summer	Fall	Winter
Apricots	Apricots	Beets	Beets
Asparagus	Avocados	Bell Peppers	Brussels Sprouts
Avocados	Beets	Broccoli	Cabbage
Cabbage	Bell Peppers	Brussels Sprouts	Collard Greens
Garlic	Berries	Cauliflower	Grapefruit
Kale	Cherries	Cranberries	Kiwifruit
Kiwifruit	Corn	Garlic	Leeks
Lettuce	Cucumbers	Grapes	Onions
Mushrooms	Eggplant	Green Beans	Oranges
Onions	Garlic	Kiwifruit	Parsnips
Peas	Green Beans	Leafy Greens	Pears
Pineapples	Mangos	Mushrooms	Pineapples
Radishes	Melons	Onions	Potatoes
Rhubarb	Peaches	Parsnips	Pumpkins
Spinach	Plums	Peas	Rutabagas
Strawberries	Summer Squash	Potatoes	Sweet Potatoes
Swiss Chard	Tomatoes	Radishes	Swiss Chard
Turnips	Watermelon	Raspberries	Turnips
	Zucchini	Yams	Winter Squash

Alkaline Superfoods

Dates	Grapes	Kale	Wild Rice
Key Limes	Melons	Mushrooms	Brazil Nuts
Mangos	Oranges	Okra	Hempseeds
Watermelons	Avocados	Olives	Walnuts
Apples	Bell Peppers	Onions	Cherries
Bananas	Cucumbers	Squash	Papayas
Berries	Ginger	Quinoa	Figs

GO SHOPPING

First things first: do not attempt shopping for groceries on an empty stomach.
Having an appropriate meal or snack
before you head out will minimize impulse buys. Bring your shopping list and
try not to stray from it!

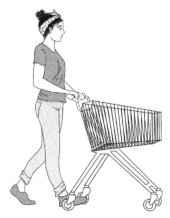

Because of blatant pesticide use, go
organic whenever available and feasible
for your income. Please reference the
dirty dozen list to see which fruits and
vegetables contain the most pesticide
residue and the clean fifteen list for best choices. Anything seasonal
within the guidelines is absolutely encouraged. If buying organic is
too expensive or not available, the next best option is certified non-
GMO. Pesticides can be prooxidant, which means they produce free
radicals in your body. Free radicals are unstable atoms that can damage cells.[71] Whether organic is available or not, I wash all my fruits
and vegetables in a sink filled with warm water, white vinegar, and a
little soap.[72]

Here are three final notes to keep in mind when shopping:

- Anything that has skin must be peeled, such as potatoes,
  cucumbers, apples, and pears (grapes are okay with skin).
  So if you are not up for peeling, you might skip these
  foods—though I sure hope you'll give them a try at least
  once!
- Only eat cooked vegetables (unless you are having a simple
  salad) during the Reset phase. This may impact what you
  choose to buy if, for example, you will only eat a certain
  veggie raw—though, again, I hope you'll be open to trying
  new approaches this week.
- If you have been diagnosed with GERD or experience a
  lot of acid reflux, stay away from fruits such as grapefruit, oranges, and tomatoes until symptoms are better
  controlled.

Shopping Checklist

FRUITS:

- ☐ Apples *(peeled)*
- ☐ Apricots
- ☐ Avocados *(let them ripen on the windowsill; ripened avocados can be stored in the refrigerator to stop the ripening process until you are ready to use them)*
- ☐ Bananas *(always a great snack; when they are ripe, cut them up and freeze for smoothies)*
- ☐ Berries *(all kinds)*
- ☐ Cherries
- ☐ Dragon fruit
- ☐ Grapefruit
- ☐ Grapes
- ☐ Guava
- ☐ Kiwi *(look for yellow kiwi also)*
- ☐ Lemons
- ☐ Limes
- ☐ Mangos
- ☐ Melons
- ☐ Oranges *(including mandarins, tangerines, clementines)*
- ☐ Papayas
- ☐ Peaches
- ☐ Pears *(peeled)*
- ☐ Persimmons

FROZEN FRUIT:

- ☐ Acai fruit packets
- ☐ Bananas *(so important for smoothies and yummy desserts)*
- ☐ Berries *(all kinds)*
- ☐ Cherries
- ☐ Cranberries
- ☐ Dragon fruit packets
- ☐ Guava
- ☐ Mangos
- ☐ Papayas
- ☐ Peaches
- ☐ Pineapple *(this might be hard on your stomach; if so, eliminate until you repair)*

DRIED FRUIT:

- ☐ Apricots
- ☐ Dates
- ☐ Figs
- ☐ Goji berries
- ☐ Mango slices
- ☐ Mulberries *(or buy fresh and dry them out in your oven—see Oven-Dried Mulberries)*

VEGETABLES:

- ☐ Artichokes
- ☐ Asparagus
- ☐ Beets
- ☐ Bell peppers
- ☐ Carrots *(cooked only)*
- ☐ Celery *(lots for juicing)*
- ☐ Cucumber
- ☐ Fennel
- ☐ Herbs *(fresh)*
- ☐ Lettuce *(soft baby lettuce, red leaf, romaine, Bibb)*
- ☐ Microgreens and sprouts
- ☐ Mung sprouts *(blanched for stir-fries and salads)*
- ☐ Mushrooms
- ☐ Onions and shallots *(cooked, and only if they are tolerated)*
- ☐ Parsnips
- ☐ Potatoes *(organic sweet potatoes, Yukon Gold, russet, white Japanese, purple)*
- ☐ Spinach
- ☐ Squash *(acorn, butternut, kabocha, spaghetti)*

Note: no cruciferous vegetables during the Reset stage *(broccoli, brussels sprouts, cauliflower)*

FROZEN VEGETABLES:

- ☐ Asparagus
- ☐ Baby greens *(spinach, microgreens, kale, Swiss, rainbow chard— see sidebar)*
- ☐ Lima beans
- ☐ Mushrooms
- ☐ Peas and carrots *(great addition to Roasted Sweet Potato Fried Rice)*
- ☐ Riced vegetables *(sweet potato—no broccoli or cauliflower till after Reset)*
- ☐ Root vegetables
- ☐ Squash *(butternut, kabocha)*

Note: no cruciferous vegetables during the Reset stage *(broccoli, brussels sprouts, cauliflower)*

All too often when loading up on healthy greens, we find ourselves with more than we can use up in a week or two. If you have an overabundance of greens or fresh herbs from your garden, grocer, or local CSA, consider freezing them to prevent food and money waste. Freezing these greens preserves their nutrients so you can use them another time, in a smoothie or as an added benefit to a dip, soup, or stew.

Greens like kale, chard, and collard greens have a thicker stem that I prefer to remove prior to freezing, but if you save them, you can later make a homemade vegetable broth. To freeze, wash and thoroughly dry the greens, then put them in a freezer bag and seal tightly, making sure there's no air. It's that simple. If a recipe calls for chopped spinach, remove it from the freezer and crunch up the greens using your hands. Instant chopped spinach!

STAPLES:

- ☐ Applesauce (unsweetened)
- ☐ Apple cider vinegar
- ☐ Avocado, olive, or coconut oil pump (oil for spraying pans and roasting veggies is minimal; remember to use parchment paper when roasting, as the paper will help cut the need for too much oil; save the healthy fats for avocados, your salad dressings, coconut milk in recipes, and olives)
- ☐ Brown or white rice flour
- ☐ Buckwheat (Cream of Buckwheat cereal, flour, whole grain)

☐ Canned coconut milk
*(a great way to fin-
ish a creamy tomato
soup instead of heavy
cream)*

☐ Canned pumpkin and
butternut squash
*(BPA-free and
non-GMO—I'll add the
pumpkin or butternut
squash to a tomato
sauce to sneak in extra
fiber or to a soup for
more depth and extra
fiber)*

☐ Coconut aminos *(this
is an excellent soy
sauce alternative;
coconut aminos have
significantly lower
sodium)*

☐ Coconut flour

☐ Coconut vinegar

☐ Dried herb blends
*(look for organic
options with no citric
acid, organic vegeta-
ble blends, Mrs. Dash
Garlic and Herb, and
lemon pepper)*

☐ Green tea *(hot or cold,
only caffeine-free)*

☐ Ground flaxseed

☐ Hemp *(hearts and
ground hempseed)*

☐ Hibiscus tea *(hot or
cold)*

☐ Honey *(raw only—raw
honey is a vital anti-
bacterial aid, great
for nausea and allergy
season)*

☐ Lemon balm tea *(hot or
cold)*

☐ Lemon and lime juice
(not from concentrate)

Hemp hearts vs. hempseeds? This may seem confusing to the first-timers reaping the benefits of
hemp. The terms are often used interchangeably,
but there is a difference. Hempseeds have a harder exterior, a soft interior, and are tougher to chew.
The hemp heart, more suited for most recipes and
easier to chew, is noticeably softer, as this is the
dehulled version of the seed.

- Maple syrup
- Nutritional yeast (a great way to add in extra B vitamins; it has a cheesy, nutty flavor and is great sprinkled on rice, potatoes, and vegetables)
- Olive oil (365 Spanish and Goya)
- Quinoa (if this causes discomfort, eliminate)
- Rice cakes
- Salsa (mild)
- Sea vegetables (dulse seaweed flakes, seaweed snacks, and Sea Seasonings brand Triple Blend Flakes)
- Tahini
- Vegetable broth
- White rice (only in moderation; organic sushi rice is sticky, quick, and easy to cook; avoid pesticides and buy organic; brown rice is too hard to digest, so avoid it for Reset)

Sea vegetables get iodine into our bodies, which is much needed if you are deficient, have sluggish thyroid issues, or are not a big fish eater. Do not take any iodine supplementation if you are on thyroid medication, as supplements can interfere with absorption issues you may already have.

DAIRY SUBSTITUTES:

- Almond milk (Three Trees or Malk)
- Coconut milk
- Flaxseed milk
- Oat milk (Malk—a great brand using organic and gluten-free oats)

JUICE:

- Aloe vera juice (George's or Lily of the Desert)
- Carrot juice (Trader Joe's or Bolthouse Farms)
- Coconut water (365 or Zico)

Unfortunately, there are not a lot of brands that carry nut milks without fillers, gums, and oils (check out foodbabe.com for a great resource that catalogs the pitfalls of additives, pesticides, fillers, and preservatives). But you can also make your own nut milks. There are many new gadgets that make creating homemade plant-based milks almost too easy—they are done in a matter of seconds with all the bells and whistles built into one appliance. And some supermarkets are starting to make this task easier while you shop, with commercial-size machines that create your own personalized combination at the push of a button. They also take care of the cleanup!

A simple and easy way to make your own plant milk at home requires just $1/2$ cup of nuts or seeds (preferably raw and organic), 4 cups of filtered water, and a pinch of salt. First, soak the nuts or seeds in filtered water for at least 4 hours or overnight. Drain, then blend them and the rest of the ingredients in a high-speed blender for about 90 seconds or until creamy and frothy. Strain (though cashews, pumpkin seeds, and hemp hearts do not need to be strained) the milk through a fine mesh nut bag over a glass bowl and store in a mason jar in the fridge for 4 to 5 days.

PREP YOUR MEALS

Spending some time preparing for your week is crucial—prep work is one of the most underrated aspects of being a chef! Most find the weekend the ideal time to get in some shopping and prep work for maximum efficiency. Here are some tips to make mealtime quick and easy.

Frozen fruits for all your smoothies are vital. If using fresh fruit, let it ripen up on your counter, then peel and freeze in chunks. Seasonal berries are great to freeze if they are starting to turn and you can't eat them fresh. Don't let the food spoil; save it for a smoothie, a bowl, or your Buckwheat Pancakes.

After a trip to the market, wash your fruits and vegetables and store them so they are ready to go. For greens, whether fresh baby spinach, salad greens, or chopped vegetables, put them in storage bags or glass containers with a paper towel to keep them crisp and extend their shelf life. For berries, I like to line a bowl or container with a paper towel and store the berries on top to keep them fresh longer.

You can also make some items ahead so you can just whip them out when it's time to eat. Make your salad dressing for the week. Get your celery ready for juicing. In a perfect world, one could make fresh juice every morning, but that might not be realistic. Consider juicing enough for two days and store it in a mason jar (or even store a portion or two in a freezable container). Precook rice and quinoa. It will keep in the fridge for a couple of days, or you can freeze some portions to use at your convenience. You will fall in love with this helpful tip. Dried fresh herbs also freeze well. And if you are making pesto (see Mixed Herb Pesto), freeze any extras for an impromptu meal, soup upgrade, or delicious addition to a salad dressing (see No-Fat Salad Dressing in a Snap). You can also clean and cut up fruit like melons or mangos and store them in a glass container in your refrigerator as a grab-and-go or snack option. The same holds for roasted vegetables—roast one or two big pans at dinnertime and you can have them for lunch the next day (see Buddha Bowls).

BUILD AWARENESS

Becoming more self-aware presents the opportunity to focus on yourself, and that's good! This proactive approach entails trial and error, though. Action, observation, and acknowledgment of positive changes will structure a new enthusiastic attitude centered around you.

Every day is a step forward. Honestly, some days you may take a step or two back, but continue to keep your eye on the prize. That's you! Becoming more aware will evolve as you become more in tune with your body. After the elimination phase, old habits like your sugar addiction won't be as appealing anymore. The new habits you establish will become just as natural as the old ones were, but with better benefits.

As you start living your life with the mindset of taking control of your health, you will realize that finding time for that goal is perfectly acceptable. Saying no to other things will be challenging at times, but it will get easier as you respect how precious your time is. In no time, you will be making conscious efforts to be better prepared, especially with meals, snacks, and even dining out. Balancing both primary and secondary food categories will always be a work in progress, as events and life are unpredictable. Learning to focus and shift your mindset will help you control your reactions. This new dynamic emphasizes how crucial becoming self-aware truly is to your health.

SET YOUR GOAL

A goal is about purpose. One cannot run to the supermarket without a list—we all know how that turns out. To achieve a goal, you need to first identify the objective. But even when we really want something, why do most of us have trouble sticking to the goals we set? Mostly this happens because there is not a concise plan of action to follow. Think of the Reset program like training for a 5K race. Finishing is a manageable and attainable goal if you properly train for it. In addition, achieving any goal involves just as much mental preparation as physical.

Take some time to consider your objective. Why did you pick up this book? Perhaps you are dealing with a chronic gastric issue. Maybe you just want to feel more energetic. Write down this intention and hang it where you'll see it daily for positive reinforcement. With that big-picture objective clearly focused in your mind, the first goal—completing the three-week Reset—will feel more achievable. Then, break down the goal into actionable steps. Your action plan is to eliminate inflammatory foods from your diet and introduce plant-based options. Everything you do from this point forward is your choice; it's your decision to make a change for the better. Your vision, commitment, and desire to succeed should push you to achieve the best possible results.

Do not underestimate your ability to see this through. Even if you keep it simple and follow the recipes and tips provided here, there may be days when you struggle. In these situations, the old you might have cruised the drive-through for something simple, easy, and manageable. This is where the mindset must change. "Mentally prepared" takes on a whole new meaning as you center the importance of your health. If you throw your arms up in the air and just can't do it, give yourself some grace. Order a healthy take-out meal, like vegetable sushi rolls with a side salad. Remember the bigger picture, do not let fear intimidate your choices, and break the impulse to go back to an unstable mindset.

Do not allow anxiety to become a barrier. It takes courage to change for the better. Be true to your goals and give hope the most significant power. When you make the most of what might seem to be a dire situation, you evolve wiser and stronger from the experience. You've got this.

Ease Your Fears When Dining Out

Dining out during the three-week Reset can be tricky, but it's not an impossible feat if there is no other alternative. Be particularly careful if you decide to dine out. When you are home and prepare your own meals, you control exactly what goes into them. Dining out does not give you that luxury.

When in the first week of Reset, you are essentially going through a detox stage. Healing immune responses and supporting your gut environment is a significant part of why certain foods are eliminated. So, should you be in a situation where you will be dining out, plan ahead and call the restaurant or check out their website online. If you make the call at a good time, say between the lunch and dinner shift, an inquiry could benefit everyone involved. Simply stating, "I need to avoid the following for health reasons," could facilitate a favorable action. In my opinion, calling ahead takes last-minute pressure off the front and back of the house and eases worry and undue anxiety during this phase.

It's also a great idea to have other options available. Packing an emergency stash of food, even a handful of dates, means you are primed for plan B if the dining experience doesn't go as anticipated. Even after Reset, make it a point to have backup choices like an apple, banana, orange, or dried fruit in your bag or car in case of an emergency. You'll thank me one day for sure.

Here are a few tips to keep in mind for navigating restaurants:

- Consider skipping gluten-free pasta, as it is probably made with corn unless someone can tell you otherwise. At times, buckwheat soba or rice noodles are available at Asian establishments.
- Think about plain rice with sautéed or steamed vegetables.
- Plain roasted or steamed potatoes with lemon are delicious. There may be some oil used when cooking; don't stress about that. Greek restaurants make the most delicious lemon potatoes. Remember to make the best of the situation.
- Choose a baked potato with avocado and a salad.
- Vegetable sushi rolls are usually available. Opt out of regular soy and see if a gluten-free version is available, or pack your coconut aminos or gluten-free tamari (tamari does contain soy).
- Before you say yes to a side of any type of sauce, remember that commercially prepared sauces are likely full of processed sugars, inflammatory fats, sodium, yeast, and preservatives.

Do not fear dining out, as healthier options are becoming more available even in the most remote areas. Remember to call ahead, be kind, and inquire accordingly. It never hurts to ask.

You are now ready for the action stage. Preparation and progress execute the plan, attention to self-care and long-term maintenance follow. Give yourself credit for making this commitment and for the steps you've taken so far.

PUT YOURSELF AT THE CENTER

Are you worthy of being front and center in your world? Without a doubt! So how come health seems to take a back seat for so many? Managing your health means giving attention to your body before it breaks down. This is the essence of being proactive—creating or controlling a situation rather than responding to it after it has happened. Being proactive with your body involves immune support, anti-inflammatory food choices, movement, and attention to how stress promotes adverse reactions.

In addition to making thoughtful food choices, you must attend to other health matters and annual screenings. What would happen if you didn't brush your teeth every day and left the damage up to the dentist at your yearly visit? Yikes. That would leave you with a painful mouth and a painful bill, both of which would have been completely preventable. Take some time now to consider what you may be putting off. Do you need to make appointments for a vision exam, doctor's visit, or dental cleaning? Preventive medicine promotes health and well-being because it raises your awareness of what's going on in your body. Happy, healthy, and fit. There's another goal worthy of your time!

SET UP YOUR SUPPORT SYSTEM

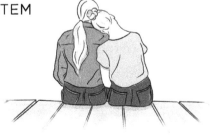

A support system begins with a close friend, coworker, gym buddy, family member, or professional who will provide you with mental, emotional, and practical support when you need it most. Likewise, they will also keep you motivated so you can knock your Reset out of the park. Find someone who will either go on this journey with you or who is willing to check in and hold you accountable.

Is asking for help something you are uncomfortable doing? Surrendering control requires courage, and seeking assistance when you need it may be the beginning of more freedom from the burden of always being in the driver's seat. When you realize you do not possess superpowers, a considerable weight is lifted. We all need some extra help, support, and love without the fear of being perceived as needy.

Asking for help or support requires open and clear communication. In my practice, I find that most of my clients just want to be heard. Breaking through those barriers is a fascinating part of what I do. Communication is underrated yet so cathartic. We cleanse thoughts, doubts, fears, and any insecurities by realizing that most of these anxieties are common yet brought on unnecessarily in everyday life situations. Self-care is a wonderful aspect of this program, so if you do not feel as though some sort of community is there for you, there may be online resources, church groups, a health coach, or an insurance benefit you overlooked that can offer support.

You will get into a routine and consistency builds confidence, but don't be afraid to ask for and accept help if you need it. Remember that solid relationships with people who will love you despite your imperfections are the ones that last the test of time.

CONSIDER PORTION SIZE

All too often, portion amounts bring about anxiety, disorders, and shame. Do we really want to carry around measuring cups and scales? What kind of message does that promote? Certainly, one of restriction or lack of control. And although we are cutting out inflammatory foods, you need not worry about how much to eat. On the Reset program, you do not have to weigh portions or count calories or carbs, but you will learn what full and satisfying means to you.

The amount of food that is considered typical and healthy is subjective, but if you feel as though you overate, you did. If, prior to Reset, you did not consistently eat various fruits and vegetables, go slowly, and eat until you are satiated. Let your brain catch up to your stomach until food choices and portions become intuitive.

We tend to overeat because much of our food choices lack sustainable nutrients. This is especially true when it comes to processed food and fast-food. With these empty calories of convenience, our bodies become hardwired to crave all the salt, sugar, and fat again and again. The addiction stems from the release of dopamine, that "feel good" hormone. This is where too much of a good thing comes into play. Although dopamine is a pleasure response, the brain can easily become overwhelmed by the bliss. The dopamine becomes too concentrated in some parts of the brain and not enough in others. This concentration is linked to poor impulse control and binge eating. So when you factor in the lack of nutrients and caloric density of processed foods and the fact that our bodies burn less energy digesting heavily processed foods, it's easy to see how eating these foods can lead to weight gain and increased metabolic risks. This holds true even in the vegan and vegetarian world where cheaply made ingredients can undo anyone's best intentions.

The goals are to relax and truly enjoy our meals—to properly nourish our brains and bodies and to learn to be more in tune when our stomachs are full.

CHAPTER 8

Week One: The Detox Stage

The first week of Reset is considered the detox stage because your body will be going through the cleansing of the unwanted waste, bacteria, and pathogens that we all accumulate. This is necessary to rid the body of inflammation. In detox, you may experience a variety of feelings such as euphoria, lightheadedness, crankiness, headaches, and possible mood swings. This is all temporary and part of the bigger picture that optimal health and its benefits bring about for those devoted to the cause. Stay focused and have patience—calm is around the corner.

GET BALANCED

CAFFEINE AND SUGAR WITHDRAWAL

Though they can be intense, caffeine headaches and the transitional withdrawal symptoms such as fatigue, irritability, and low energy are short lived. Other unpleasant detox complaints are anxiety and muscle aches. Sugar withdrawal symptoms present as headaches and feelings of sluggishness, moodiness, and anxiety. Keep in mind that cutting back on the sweet stuff will pay off soon enough. Identify these common signs, know they are temporary, get plenty of rest, avoid stress, and in no time, you will be over this hump. Remind yourself why you are participating in Reset and stay motivated to eliminate the inflammation. Fuel yourself with whole-food alternatives like fresh fruit and fiber-rich foods to combat these unhealthy cravings. Stay hydrated, as dehydration contributes to sugar cravings.

REST AND DIGEST

Two critical components of proper immune support are resting and digesting. Remind yourself frequently of the importance of appropriate digestive functions. When we do not eat consciously, we do not digest properly. You will not digest your food appropriately—and your body will therefore not reap its full benefits—if you are stressed or upset while eating, eating on the run, or distracted by the TV or something else. This kind of disrupted eating sets off adverse reactions throughout the body, like food sensitivities or intolerances. Compromised immune health becomes a significant part of illness if not addressed and supported with a healthful attitude.

Aim to be in a restorative parasympathetic state when you eat. This means eating while calm and stress-free. Emphasizing how vital the parasympathetic state is at mealtime means you'll become more conscious as well. In situations of stress, the digestive process is limited, meaning effective swallowing, the release of digestive enzymes, and proper blood and oxygen flow to the stomach are negatively affected. When we have these altered metabolic responses, the body works longer and harder to process things like sugar and fat in the blood. When our metabolism is overworked, we are at increased risk of inflammatory and autoimmune diseases. Practice enjoying your meals slowly and deliberately to keep digestion optimal.

EXPECT MORE ELIMINATION

As you bring more alkalinity back to your body, you will notice that you are eliminating more than usual. Yes, I mean your bowels. Eliminating waste is excellent and expected as you are flushing your colon of impurities and old food. You are improving circulation in the intestines and getting things going. You will notice less constipation, bloating, and puffiness.

If you have been constipated, you may notice that things are beginning to move along in your intestines. You may experience mild cramping or nausea along with the need to eliminate. The first week is different for everyone, but typically most clients feel they are getting cleaned out. This is good and expected.

On the other hand, if you were diagnosed with something like SIBO, *H. pylori*, IBS, or leaky gut, your stools before Reset might have been watery and not well formed. You should notice that you are eliminating a lot in Reset, but also that the stool is better formed and not as watery. See the Bristol Stool Scale from chapter 1 for reference.

BE AWARE

TRY A LOVING-KINDNESS MEDITATION

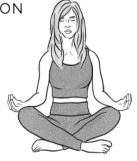

As you know, stress is a main cause of inflammation. So if your stress level runs high most days, it's important to find ways to minimize it during Reset to maximize healing. High stress levels increase blood pressure, and that pressure damages blood vessels and inflates the likeliness of blockages and heart attacks. Other common effects of stress include anxiety, restlessness, and lack of motivation. Less stressful responses promote positive changes to heart rate and blood pressure, not to mention dozens of other physical and behavioral benefits.

One effective way to reduce stress is with meditation. One of the simplest meditations out there is a mindful meditation known as loving-kindness meditation. This practice comes from Buddhist teachings, though the specific one I adapted was developed by Jon Kabat-Zinn. His lifelong research concerns the effectiveness of stress reduction through mindfulness meditation. He also correlates how stress negatively affects cognitive emotions and the immune system.

This meditation emphasizes the importance of living in the moment. Gestures of kindness, whether to yourself or to others, also generate the release of the hormone oxytocin, which pushes the fight-or-flight response into a mode that is more rested and relaxed.

The world is harsh at times, and a little compassion for yourself may change your mindset to a more healthful one. This meditation can also send positive thoughts and understanding to a loved one. Why not? Genuine human connection is as essential as the air we breathe. With daily affirmations, if we profess the importance of what we need, how we want to be seen, and why it's important to love us for who we truly are, our value grows. Encouraging words directed toward another are a supportive morale booster that may trigger a positive change. We all know too well that positive shifts need to come from within, but if you modify your behaviors and continue daily affirmations, you may succeed in improving relationships, even when another is in denial or flat out refuses your best intentions. We all need a little more love and kindness in our lives and in the world. Positive affirmations may also help overcome self-sabotaging and negative thoughts.

All you have to do is repeat the following two times:

> May I be happy.
> May I be well.
> May I be healthy.
> May I be safe.
> May I be loved.

That is all. Simply close your eyes and say these words to yourself whenever you need support. You will notice how your breathing slows and your worries seem less important.

PRIORITIZE YOURSELF

Let's not forget self-care and the benefits of finding time to focus on what makes you happy. Do not confuse self-care with being selfish. Selfishness excludes and takes from others, whereas self-care is about recharging your battery without depleting someone else's.

When you take responsibility for yourself, you can care for others without resentment.

Be gentle with yourself, as self-care should not be a burden. The effort feels good on some days and not so realistic on others. Do not let shame get the best of you, as shame comes with a dark cloud of negativity. Set up realistic and uncomplicated expectations of what makes you feel happy. What self-care looks like can vary: a hobby, an exercise class that leaves you feeling energized and proud, continuing education, a haircut, new sheets, good hygiene, hydration, a hot bath, or simply taking your full lunch break. Even something as uncomplicated as a short daily walk is excellent self-care; not only do you get fresh air and vitamin D, but walking aids digestion. The benefits are motivating and empowering.

In Reset, it is advisable to avoid high-impact exercise. While exercise promotes blood circulation and the release of toxins, too much of a good thing could boomerang on those precious hormones we are trying to balance. Too much impact is difficult for the digestive system to handle during this transitional period. Low-impact physical activity, on the other hand, is safe and encouraged. Anything that does not push your limits—a daily walk, Pilates, a gentle yoga class—is desirable and prudent for optimal results.

All in moderation holds true in most aspects of a balanced life. Smile more, show kindness, and turn negative into positive. Anything rewarding that stimulates happy hormonal responses in our brains is a win-win, linking pleasure, happiness, and a clearer path forward.

PREPARE FOR POTENTIAL OVERWHELM

Any new situation or routine can potentially overwhelm you. Soon enough, this will pass as you process this unfamiliar journey, initiate self-care, and balance your footing in this new world of better health.

You may find in situations of overwhelm that redirecting your attention or emotions to what you can control helps. Shift your focus away from the uncontrollable, take a break, breathe, and remind yourself that feeling overwhelmed is usually temporary. You will be in the honeymoon stage soon enough!

When coping feels out of your control, speak with a mental health professional.

STAY EDUCATED

KEEP IT SIMPLE

In the first week, as you clear your body of inflammatory foods, re-member, it is still adjusting. The fiber in plant-based foods promotes the growth of healthy bacteria. As we rid the body of impurities, it is not uncommon to feel unwell or a little gassy or crampy after a meal. Remember, as optimal food choices cleanse, they are also encourag-ing the growth of good bacteria through fermentation. Both those soluble and insoluble fibers are working simultaneously to demo and then rebuild a solid foundation in your near future. That short-term agitation will subside as cleansing alters the microbiome to heal and adapt. Too often, diets lacking adequate fiber (those that are high in dairy, eggs, and animal protein) can stimulate an increase in disease-promoting bacteria. Embrace this healing stage and this newfound balance within.

Keeping life simple in this stage is vital.

BENEFITS OF YOUR NEW MORNING RITUALS

Celery Juice

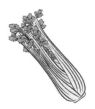

Celery juice is the perfect electrolyte next to coco-nut water. It is so important to keep your body hy-drated and cooled, and drinking celery juice is a great habit to continue beyond the Reset phase. Celery is rich in phytonutrient antioxidants that contain anti-inflammatory properties. In addition, it has been used for its antifungal and antibacterial effects since ancient times.[73] It also contains calcium, silicon, and vitamin K to aid in strengthening bones. The healing prop-erties in celery juice reduce acidity and bring a more alkaline state as well as aiding in the proper digestion of what you eat throughout the day. Not only will the juice improve digestion, the salts, minerals, and fiber pick up bacteria, pathogens, and excess cholesterol compounds in the gut and push them out in the elimination process.

Most of us overwork and inflame our organs either by eating the wrong foods, experiencing consistent stress, or taking medications for a prolonged period of time. When there is an imbalance in our gut health, the stomach lining becomes compromised. Celery juice can significantly replenish depleted levels of gastric mucus. This mucus coating is an essential part of your esophagus and is needed to prevent ulcers and acid reflux. If we do not have a resilient lining in our stomachs, we open the door for immune reactions, leaky gut, undigested foods fermenting, and the possibility of chronic illnesses.

Do not add ginger, lemon, or apples, as anything added will take away from its health benefits. Lastly, celery is on the dirty dozen list, meaning it is on the list of vegetables that pick up the most pesticides. For that reason, buy organic.

Lemon Water

Maintaining proper pH balance in your body coincides with good microbiome (gut) harmony. Warm water and lemon acts as a detoxifying agent and aids in maintaining good digestive health.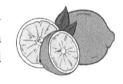

In our bodies, lemons in their natural state are acidic, with a pH of about 2 (very acidic). Once metabolized and thoroughly digested, lemons become alkaline with a pH well above 7 (alkaline). Small amounts daily are optimal. It is also a rich source of vitamin C, cleanses internal waste, removes toxins to support immune system deficiencies, and stimulates colon health, acting as a laxative for some. It's simple and a morning ritual that most enjoy.

Energy Fruit Smoothie

Aloe vera juice has been used medicinally for centuries. The juice comes from the aloe vera plant, and historically, it has been used both topically and orally. High in polyphenols, it boosts many antioxidant-rich compounds that aid in reducing inflammation, especially within our digestive tract. In addition, it helps with lowering blood sugar levels. The juice can be bought bottled, but look for 100 percent aloe vera juice preferably from the whole leaf. Making your own may require some time, but when you see the large leaves for sale at your supermarket, the process only requires skinning the leaf like you would a fish and pulverizing the aloe vera gel in a blender for all those medicinal benefits.

Bananas are very low in saturated fat, cholesterol, and sodium. They are a good source of dietary fiber, vitamin C, vitamin B6, potassium, and manganese. Your best bet when shopping for bananas is bright-yellow and slightly freckled fruit. If you are going to eat them in the next several days, this is the time when they are ripe, easy to peel, and sweet and tender.

Blueberries (especially wild blueberries) are the number one powerhouse of nutrients. High in polyphenols and prebiotic fiber, berries help break the sugar craving cycle in addition to giving your cells instant energy without raising your insulin levels drastically. In addition, pigments of berries (strawberries, mulberries, raspberries, and blackberries) provide essential amino acids and impressive antioxidants straight from Mother Earth. Most wild blueberries grow in Maine and Canada, so unless you're lucky enough to harvest these tiny powerhouse treats, go to the freezer section of your supermarket and stock up!

Coconut water is rich in dietary fiber, enzymes, vitamin C, minerals, and amino acids. On the flip side, it is low in calories, chlorides, and cholesterol. Coconut water helps speed up your metabolism and creates a feeling of fullness.

Drinking coconut water will keep your skin hydrated and balance its pH levels. Applying the water directly to your skin is said to reduce acne; lessen visible signs of aging, stretch marks, and cellulite; and even treat eczema. Drinking coconut water will also help boost your immune system and fight the common cold and flu, thus keeping your cardiovascular health in top shape. It's always best consumed cold!

Cilantro stimulates the gut and aids in the production of stomach acid. It is also beneficial for indigestion, constipation, and gas. Getting lots of this herb into your routine helps eliminate heavy metals and unwanted bacteria from your body. When picking cilantro, bright green is the way to go; avoid bunches that are starting to brown. Don't forget about the stems, they offer just as much flavor and nutrients. Fresh cilantro tends to hold on to dirt, so wash this incredibly vibrant and tasty herb thoroughly.

Ground hempseed contains all nine essential amino acids and its protein composition is similar to an egg white (ideal for muscle recovery) but with the benefits of more fiber, calcium, iron, and healthy fats. Rich in omega-3 fatty acids to protect heart and brain functions, it is also wonderful to sprinkle on hot cereals and yogurt after Reset.

Mango is the "king of fruits," as it has a long list of overall health benefits. Mangos contain large doses of vitamin C and vitamin A. They are considered an alkaline fruit, which means they help balance the acid we carry in our digestive tracts. Select mangos that are firm and bright with a distinct pleasant aroma and avoid any with black or soft spots.

Pineapple is a tasty addition to any smoothie. Pineapple is an excellent source of the trace mineral manganese, an essential cofactor in several enzymes important in energy production and antioxidant defenses. Its vitamins and minerals act as a natural anti-inflammatory agent and support the immune system and digestive tract. Picking the ideal pineapple is easy if you remember this: for optimal ripeness, the shell should be firm but slightly soft when you squeeze.

Spinach tops the charts in nutrient richness. It offers twice as much fiber as other greens and is a decent source of iron and protein. Like other dark greens, spinach is an excellent source of beta-carotene, a powerful disease-fighting antioxidant. A diet rich in antioxidants helps reduce the risk of developing cataracts, heart disease, and cancer. Spinach is one of the dirty dozen foods, so buy organic to get the most out of spinach's health benefits.

THE INNER WORKINGS OF INSULIN

During the digestion of certain foods, insulin, a hormone, is released by the pancreas. Insulin controls how much glucose (energy) is in your blood. Insulin then aids in the transport of glucose into the body's cells. The liver and muscles store the excess energy as either glycogen (short-term storage) or triglycerides in fatty cells. Triglycerides are later released for energy in between meals.

Depending on the size and content of the meal, your blood glucose should respond by slightly rising. Insulin then makes its way from the pancreas into the blood. This energy (our food supply) moves into our cells and metabolizes when we give our bodies the right foods. With better choices, blood sugar and insulin levels in our blood slow and stop until we need the energy again. Insulin resistance, on the other hand, appears when there is excess glucose (sugar) in the blood that's not getting transported to the cells effectively, which leads to inflammation.

The primary purpose of insulin is compromised if driving through Chick-fil-A or other fast-food spots several times a week is your jam. When we feed our bodies the wrong carbs (white flour, refined sugars, and processed foods), our muscles, fat, and liver cells don't respond well, so more insulin is released. This resistance can quickly become a vicious cycle.

Eating fruit in the morning (during Reset) gives you instant energy, satiates your hunger, and digests quickly without stress to the stomach lining. With this protocol, you provide your cells with the energy they need. You are also giving your liver and other organs a much-needed break.

If your gut is compromised and you eat something like oatmeal with almonds and blueberries, proper conversion of energy to cells is insufficiently handled on account of the present irritation. We need efficient energy and healing from the easily absorbed foods during this phase of Reset. Fat and protein—even from healthy foods—potentially increase inflammation, so we lessen the load during the healing phase. Even the most active and disciplined eaters can hold on to excess weight in the form of bloating from toxins, undigested foods, and an imbalance of harmful bacteria in the gut. Sound familiar?

Also contemplate eating smaller meals more frequently for less of an overload on your precious organs. The Reset protocol also adequately feeds and calms the adrenals to help these organs perform more efficiently. Our adrenal glands play a dominant role in stress, the release of too much cortisol, and subsequently, the release of even more insulin as an adrenal response from the liver, where excess glucose is stored. Mindful fiber-rich choices manage your blood sugar with proper insulin distribution.

The right combinations of plant-based foods eaten at the correct times will fuel the cells, detoxify, and aid in the elimination of existing irritation. In addition, the resistant starch in fiber-rich foods help make our cells more responsive to insulin. The benefits of these outlined choices include regulating blood sugar, phasing out that constant craving for food, and providing essential amino acids, vitamins, minerals, and more alkalinity to the body.

CHAPTER 9

Week Two: The Honeymoon Stage

In the honeymoon stage, you start to settle in and become familiar with your new routine. Week two is the wonderful feeling of excitement where you think, *This new routine could really grow on me,* and you are eager as your relationship with self-care grows, blossoms, and holds the promise of only better changes coming your way.

GET BALANCED

SUPPORT ENDOCRINE HEALTH

Going into your second week of Reset, you have abolished most simple carbohydrates, the biggest disruptors of your endocrine system. Simple carbs without rich micronutrients include milk or milk products and processed and refined sugars such as candy, cookies, table sugar, syrups, and soft drinks. The glucose that we get from processed and refined foods is frequently stored as fat. Elimination of these inflammatory foods will have you feeling lighter in the second week.

Figuring out what works exceptionally well for your body is an intrinsic aspect of Reset. Many people think low-carb diets are supposed to work more efficiently on a nutritional level, but too few fiber-rich carbohydrates negatively impact thyroid function and can cause muscle cramping and fatigue. As hormones are fundamental to all the systems in our bodies, removing the highly processed and refined foods resolves the issue without disrupting this precious balance any further. Seventy percent of the foods found on supermarket shelves contain genetically modified ingredients. Other hormone disruptors include those found in lower quality animal protein, dairy, cleaning products, shampoos, body creams, and air fresheners.

Another big offender is the soy industry. The ingredients are typically heavily modified isolated proteins, soy isoflavone supplements, and foods made with textured vegetable protein (protein powders and nutrition bars). After Reset, you may reintroduce pure soy products such as tofu, edamame, miso, and tempeh, but avoid the rest.

ENJOY YOUR NEWFOUND ENERGY

As you eliminate these inflammatory foods, you typically feel lighter as the new week progresses. The complex, whole-food carbs you are eating are less likely to be stored as fat, and you will notice you have more energy, a better attitude, more quality sleep, happiness, and less stress. Make note—it may be subtle or you may feel super energetic. This is all normal and very good!

CATCH THE CURVEBALLS

Never attach guilt and shame to food. The reasoning behind the 10 percent window is that you don't always have to be perfect. Having an ideal setup is impossible, no matter how committed and passionate you are about feeling your best. We all have fires to put out, unexpected distractions, and circumstances we don't anticipate that can throw off the best intentions for a healthy meal. Navigating these scenarios without too much stress becomes more manageable as you build your foundation.

The best-case outcomes happen when you are prepared for hurdles.

If your mealtime doesn't unfold as you expected, let it go and move to plan B. Backup plans might include having soups or a batch of pancakes in the freezer. Save take-out menus from restaurants that offer healthy or more customizable options. Be okay with compromise and throw guilt out the window! Catch that curveball, minimize the stress response, and have some contingency plans in place.

BE AWARE

TRY THE SMILE MEDITATION

Who doesn't have time for a ten-minute meditation? I recommend the Inner Smile Meditation by Qigong master Lee Holden (find the link in the Resources section). This is hands down my favorite meditation. It uses the visualization of a golden light to wash away old, cloudy gray energy; through breathing exercises, you inhale a clarifying light and vibration-type smile energy to cleanse the entire body. Tension, knots, and muscles are in for a treat! His therapeutic voice does the trick, and when there is no time to sit and close your eyes, play it in the car while you're driving for the simple reason that it is relaxing. It sure beats the news.

GO FOR A WALK

Walking is one of the best ways to improve and maintain essential activity on this new journey. Just thirty minutes a day can strengthen bones, reduce excess fat, and build muscle and endurance. Other numerous benefits include heart health, low-impact fitness, increased circulation, better sleep, cognitive support, and the natural release of endorphins. Plus, it's free!

TAKE A NAP

A short twenty- to thirty-minute nap may sound silly, but if time allows, why not try it out? A brief nap can do wonders to improve mood, sharpen focus, and reduce fatigue. It's not recommended daily, but more for those days when you feel especially tired. It could be just the much-needed rest and subsequent burst of energy your body is looking for.

If you are someone who has trouble sleeping throughout the night, daytime naps may not be for you.

ENHANCE YOUR SLEEP HYGIENE

Improving and maintaining healthy sleep habits is essential for good health and an important part of Reset. Whether you are unable to fall or remain asleep or if waking up too early is something you can relate to, the following 101 on sleep patterns is here to help.

When we sleep, we allow our body to rest, heal, grow, and repair. Disruptive situations such as travel, stress, changes in schedules or eating habits, or any type of conflict can cause struggle when all we want is a restful night. Without consistent sleep patterns, our brains have difficulty resetting, our hormones are compromised, and the imbalance affects concentration, anxiety, pain, sickness, and many other mood concerns.

Lack of sleep affects the following hormones:

Cortisol: Although cortisol is often thought to be released in stressful situations, our levels of cortisol are also naturally highest in the mornings to help us start the day. An overabundance of cortisol (from stress) affects when and how this vital hormone does its job and hinders the ability to produce melatonin.

Melatonin: Melatonin regulates the circadian rhythm in our bodies. As the light darkens and we prepare to sleep, our brain naturally releases this hormone. Normal rhythms are negatively affected with bright lights and electronics, so something as simple as dimming the lights at night and keeping electronic use to a minimum will boost this hormone. Current research on light and its vital role to our circadian rhythm suggests that light, even the lack of it, affects our melatonin production as we prepare for sleep. There are different theories on what kind of light is best for the sleep-wake cycle, but the dominant theory is that melatonin suppression occurs more with bright lights. My suggestion is to create the most relaxing mood with lighting as you prepare for bedtime. Overhead lights and bright wall lighting with cooler tones promote wakefulness and a more focused attitude. Save that mood lighting for another time. If you want to relax, try low over-head lighting with warm color tones for a calm, relaxing, cozy, and more sleepy environment.

Growth hormone (GH): This hormone stimulates growth, cell re-production, and cell regeneration. Supporting this hormone naturally requires regular movement, a reduction in processed foods and sugars, and healthy sleep patterns.

Gamma-aminobutyric acid (GABA): The critical release of this restorative hormone allows us to relax and facilitates the function of the nerve cells to communicate. Deep breathing, yoga, and medita-tion stimulate it. Remember also that food impacts mood. Many of the foods you are consuming in Reset naturally stimulate this hormone. On the other hand, drugs, alcohol, and processed foods decrease GABA production.

When your mind is calm, your cortisol drops and stress disap-pears. With lifestyle modifications, balancing your body's chemistry will bring symmetry to your hormones. Create a peaceful atmosphere in your bedroom with clean sheets, no clutter, and drawn shades to enhance and stimulate this natural therapeutic process.

PRACTICE SAYING NO

The art of saying no teaches you to appreciate yourself and your valu-able time. Are your need-to-do lists and want-to-do lists causing anger, hurt, and bitterness in your life?

For example, if your growth, spirit, or health is compromised be-cause you have a hard time saying no or asking for help, and you feel ob-ligated to work late, join that friend, or babysit again for your neighbor, that would be a red flag. If you become angry at your partner, kids, or ev-eryone at the supermarket with little provocation, that behavior would be considered distressing. If saying yes all the time has turned you into a stressed-out, moody, and resentful person, it may be time to reevaluate.

You need to give yourself time to realign, reexamine, reestablish, nourish properly, and enjoy life. To do this, sometimes you have to say no. We all need to fulfill obligations, but take a step back and see what is really necessary. When your full capacity is restored, you can get to the need-tos because you want to.

STAY EDUCATED

READ LABELS

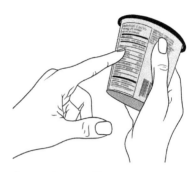

Becoming a label reader and questioning additives may lead to answers about
nagging symptoms you cannot resolve,
such as migraines or a chronic runny
nose. It could be that most of us are not
immediately affected by additives, but
are we slowly putting ourselves in danger down the road?

No matter how an ingredient presents, its origin should be ques-
tioned, as our body has to recognize and break it down. Disruptions to
the established bacteria are frequently associated with inflammation
from unrecognized foods, additives, and preservatives.[74] Somehow,
these processed ingredients must add up eventually in whatever quantity we consume. Food for thought, indeed.

This is where label reading comes in. First, keep in mind that the
first three ingredients make up the largest part of what you're eating.
Look for the best quality, simplest ingredients and avoid products that
start with added sugars or artificial sweeteners, inflammatory oils,
processed soy, refined flours, thickeners, stabilizers, and emulsifiers.
You may be surprised by how many packaged foods, sports drinks, and
protein powders—and also cosmetics and pharmaceuticals—contain
hidden added sugars. If a packaged food contains more than eight to
ten ingredients, pass it by.

Big companies use many loopholes to bypass prohibitions against
including additives and chemicals in our convenience foods. Foodbabe.
com is a wonderful, eye-opening source on what happens under the
nose of the Food and Drug Administration (FDA).

Next, dietary fiber, fat, protein, sodium, and sugar content offer
essential information. Choosing foods that will keep you feeling fuller
longer is more important than their calorie content. Calories are relevant, but not the end-all, be-all. Serving sizes are also important to note,
as some products give nutritional values based on a two-serving size.

The bottom line is that it's time to put confidence into what you
can control. Getting the best idea of what's in your food is a work in

progress. A good mantra to take to the grocery store is "If I can't say it, I won't eat it." If you don't know what it is, why put it into your body? Put some quality time into making the best nutritional choices.

Learning more about what's in your food might have you questioning why there are so many inflammatory oils, sugars, and preservatives in products. Your addiction to potato chips may be just that. It's not the potato, it's the high temperature frying in subpar oils with salts, additives, and addictive preservatives. Do not fall prey to a clever logo or marketing phrasing, as many touted benefits are not supported by science.

In the Reset phase, the focus is on fresh, whole foods, so you won't be purchasing many packaged items. But convenience items are just that—convenient—and we all need to purchase them on occasion. Get into the habit now of looking at labels and considering what is actually in the foods you are buying. When you get into the Maintenance phase, the section Becoming a Confident Label Reader will offer more specific ways to make positive choices with prepackaged products.

WATCH FOR HIDDEN SUGAR

Sugar is hidden everywhere. Big companies make considerable amounts of money tricking their consumers into thinking "natural flavors" are beneficial. Processed sugar, sugar substitutes, and alcohol-derived sugar alternatives wreak havoc on our microbiome, cause inflammation, and compromise our immune system. Aside from the basic names we know as sugar, be aware that there are close to two hundred pseudo names for sugar on ingredient lists. Anything ending in "ose" is sugar. Other deceiving manufactured code words are cane, nectar, and syrup.

There are good sources of sugar, such as pure maple syrup from trees—which offers benefits of naturally occurring vitamins and minerals—and honey from bees. Pick the most natural and nutritional sources and remember, all in moderation.

CHAPTER 10

Week Three: The Transformation Stage

By the time you get to week three, your gut intuition is sharper. You are more in tune with your body's wants and needs. The right carbs, protein, and fats will help distribute energy efficiently, but this composition differs from person to person. Factors like a balanced gut environment, diet, sleep, stress, home environment, and your unique genetics are vital information. You are still developing your ideal path, so remember to take it one day at a time.

GET BALANCED

HEALTHY RELATIONSHIPS

According to Brené Brown, vulnerability should be "our most accurate measure of courage." In a healthy relationship, we must make ourselves vulnerable in order to trust, openly communicate, listen, be intimate, and work through disagreements. Having thriving relationships is also a big part of your circle of life because all these little pieces of well-being are essential for balance.

In any relationship we welcome into our lives, we courageously hope for the best and make ourselves vulnerable for the most favorable outcome. We want supportive and sustainable friendships, marriages, and work relationships that thrive from the effort and compromise it takes to make them work.

Knowing when to show up is a supportive measure that gives value to any relationship, but if you are always the one who is present and you often feel as though you are on this path alone, it may be time to reevaluate the strength of that bond. Toxic bonds show a pattern of disrespect, controlling behaviors, resentment, jealousy, violence, unpleasant communication, and lack of support. We cannot get along with everyone and must pick our battles and be aware of our own defensiveness in times of conflict. But if you feel drained, intimidated, exhausted, and afraid in any relationship, determine if that is supporting you or drowning your efforts.

A very dear friend of mine often says, "When someone shows you who they are, believe them the first time." As I get older, I look for quality above quantity when it comes to relationships. Trust your gut on this one and believe in yourself first. When you are a good friend, listener, and companion, you deserve to get what you give.

CLEANING UP THE CLUTTER

There are two kinds of clutter: physical and mental. Beginning with physical clutter, think about things you may have put on the back burner. That project may be starting a vegetable garden or flower bed, painting a room, or donating or getting rid of stuff you no longer need or are tired of looking at. Decluttering offers health related benefits. Chances are, when you clean your home, you will be removing potential environmental allergens, alleviating the stress and anxiety clutter causes, and hopefully sleeping better because you have physically and mentally accomplished something.

In considering mental clutter, go back to your Circle of Life diagram and track your progress. Determine what needs work and commit to the growth process in every way that offers value. For example, if your spirituality needs work, figure out how that aspect of your life could use improvements. When we choose the path that holds the most faith, gratitude, and love, incorporating those practices into our daily lives is often hindered by events such as a global pandemic. Detours from those core values happen to the best of us. Getting back on track to enhance that part of your life could involve spiritual readings, going back to church, or attending synagogue. Spending time in nature, meditation, finding free networks of support, and even mindful breathing practices are other ways to invite spirituality back into your life for more balance.

Disorder affects everyone, and undue stress can strain relationships. Figure out a project that can cultivate a cleaner, clutter-free environment and strengthen your mind and spirit.

BE AWARE

KISS THOSE CRAVINGS GOODBYE

One of the best aspects of Reset is the ability to squash cravings. Cravings are usually a symptom of a nutrition deficiency or a stress trigger. An undesirable habit can become ancient history in the three-week elimination phase. Through the process of crowding out those inflammatory choices by introducing better alternatives, you are creating a more favorable habit. Whatever pushed you in the direction of unhealthy choices is becoming a thing of the past, so it's time to kiss those cravings goodbye.

Now, let's reflect on what may push you in the direction of habitually reaching for sweets, such as grabbing a bowl of ice cream every night after dinner. It might be a good time to search the ingredient label for unfavorable added ingredients now that you are more in tune with how your body is feeling. It could be a habit or an effective distraction from unresolved emotions. Some use drugs to soothe, others use food. Connecting with more balance in all areas of your life will support emotional responses. By calming our body and minds, we can take a deeper look into which areas we struggle with most and if food is used to soothe or even punish.

We are creatures of habit. Most of us like rituals and structure, but as you Reset, you have decided those old habits do not serve you well. By building a new foundation and filling up on more nutritious meals, one loses the yearning for those addictive treats. You have reinforced that energy with dedication to make sustainable improved choices. Rewiring your brain is not only physical but also involves the psychological process of using food emotionally. Is food a distraction, emotional response, or reward? As you learn about the consequences of making less than healthy choices both on and off the plate, old habits will die off and a more desirable mindset will sidestep the desire to walk down the candy aisle on your next visit to the grocery store.

REVISIT YOUR GOALS

When you look back at this journey, revisit how you felt as you began this exploration of your health goals. Though it's excellent to celebrate when you reach your destination, reflecting on the journey and remembering your small struggles and successes helps solidify your intent. Life never unfolds perfectly as planned, but you are now better equipped to self-advocate, set new goals, and maintain a solid foundation.

This may be a great time to go back to those original goals you wrote down and appreciate the dedication and attention you gave to self-care. In addition, you could certainly tweak those goals or create new ones. At times, thoughtful reflection uncovers new values and objectives, which are all worth exploring to make progress in any aspect of your life.

Commit to yourself and your health. Acknowledge and recover from roadblocks. Value your good intentions—whether good or bad, those bumps in the road are a learning experience. An attainable course of action involves goals, a plan, progress check-ins, and an open-minded perspective that nothing will ever be perfect.

MAKE NOTE OF POSITIVE CHANGES

As this adventure unfolds for you, figuring out what healthy means for you is also a critical part of this journey. Moving forward into the Maintenance phase, please stay positive with the following:

Moderation: Eating in response to emotions, whether negative or positive, is okay and part of enjoying life, but the emotional side of indulging *all the time* can move us away from self-nourishment.

Flexibility around food choices: It's not about being on or off track when traveling or eating out; it's about adopting a way of eating that aligns with your values and circumstances. Be the oddball. You will look and feel so good, everyone will want to know your secret.

Variation: It's perfectly healthy and encouraged to deviate from the foods you usually eat. Mixing it up with different fruits and vegetables is a more rounded way of eating, plus you will keep your metabolism working at its most efficient.

Beliefs around food: Don't categorize food as good or bad. That attaches guilt and shame to them. When you're out with friends, enjoy the company you're with instead of focusing on the food you eat.

Breathing: Did you know that when you inhale, you should push your belly out? Most of us breathe through our chest when, in fact, a *real* breath should come from our stomach. On the exhale, bring your belly in.

STAY EDUCATED

REFLECTING ON YOUR JOURNEY

Spend some time reflecting on the last three weeks, making note of symptoms that have either subsided or lessened considerably as a result of eliminating inflammatory foods. Any sort of positive change is a significant accomplishment, and along with your new mindset and awareness, it is your new foundation.

As you enter your Maintenance phase, enjoy your better choices, and dismiss guilt or judgment if that doesn't always happen. Remember to rest and digest. Aim to thoroughly chew, appreciate, and enjoy your food in a relaxed state of mind. Watch the labels on convenience foods and continue focusing on a plant-based whole-food diet. In addition, be more aware of what affects your body, moods, and overall well-being. Every little thing you do, hold on to, and obsess over will affect your health. Let it all go at the end of the day. Don't let those little things hold you back from something great.

Review your Circle of Life diagram often and aim to balance it out. For example, we cannot choose how others act, but how we react will determine our stress levels. You have given yourself a gift and are more aware of how your body responds to secondary foods, which is good news for your primary foods goal list. I encourage you to look back and acknowledge and celebrate your accomplishments.

If you stay in the Reset phase a little longer (see Am I Ready for the Maintenance Phase? in part 3), I recommend finding more time for self-care acts that make you happy and relax your mind and spirit. Remember those goals, remind yourself of those triumphs, and celebrate by practicing uninterrupted new lifestyle choices.

PART THREE

_____

Maintenance

You have arrived at part 3. Congratulations for accomplishing so much in the past three weeks! We all take something different from this experience—perhaps you found hydrating more helps you feel better. Maybe you've found new plant-based options that you love or realized that self-care is a doable and significant part of your well-being. But perhaps the biggest change is that your gut is more balanced and your inflammation levels have subsided. This is all great and to be expected. You are moving from one plateau to the next and are hopefully feeling more energized with fewer digestion issues. Maybe you are feeling more emotionally balanced and finding it easier to ditch any poor habits. If you are—and even if you're not there yet, as everybody recalibrates at their own pace—make note of this progress and celebrate it.

In part 3, we will cover everything you need to know about reintroducing eliminated foods. I can't stress enough how important it is to do this gradually. Remind yourself that you started this program because diets failed you, your digestion was abnormal, inflammation of the gut was causing a lot of discomfort, or any other reason. Don't rush to jump back in! You are still on a journey. Now that you've begun the healing process, reintroduce foods in small steps.

We will focus on the following topics:

- Looking out for signs that you may need to stay in Reset a while longer
- Determining what Maintenance will look like for you, specifically by making informed food choices
- Getting informed about common health concerns and considerations related to the link between food, cognitive functions, and a stabilized gut microbiome
- Trying more plant-based recipes that support your health
- Supporting your new gut environment by maintaining beneficial bacteria and continuing to build a robust immune system
- Reinforcing the solid foundation you have built in the last three weeks
- Fine-tuning your balanced plates, self-care, and your new mindset

CHAPTER 11

I Finished Reset 90/10. Now What?

Now that Reset is complete, you can reintroduce eliminated foods!

Well, maybe not all of them, but certainly more vegetables, grains, legumes, nuts, and seeds. But before you start, it's time to reflect on the past three weeks. Acknowledge that you've become more aware of what affects your body, moods, and overall well-being. This is a massive step toward feeling your best from this point forward because a greater awareness of foods, meal prep, and eating helps you make wise choices not just with food but with other aspects of your life. You have personally witnessed the positive results a plant-based shift can bring. You understand the effort in creating harmony both on and off the plate.

Now you can expand your food options. A step-by-step approach is best, so you can keep track of what's working and what may still be contributing to inflammation. You will also benefit from understanding more about whole-body functionality, as well as important health considerations. So please don't skip to the recipes just yet. It's time to further explore what building your foundation looks like for you specifically.

AM I READY FOR THE MAINTENANCE PHASE?

For most bodies, a three-week elimination program is enough to decrease inflammation significantly, reduce bloating and gas, increase your energy level and cognitive clarity, and balance cravings. You've created a healthy foundation that is yours specifically. Remember your goals: Have you ditched the sugar habit and are you ready to denounce most processed foods? If yes, and if you feel great and are ready to diversify with more plant-based options, you're probably ready for Maintenance!

This phase is called "Maintenance" because you've made the commitment to keep digestive processes running smoothly from here on out, and paved the way for benefits to keep pouring in—it is the sustainable action of keeping all your best efforts going with enhancements on what you've learned already. You are moving on to the reinoculate-and-repair stage of this mission. You have created more stability by removing potentially harmful triggers and given much attention to the overall health of the host of this party. Remember, gut habitat has a profound influence on many everyday functions.

In Maintenance, we expand on the foundation and reintroduce some eliminated food groups one by one, paying attention to your body's responses. With all the new recipes Maintenance offers, developing and broadening ways to incorporate more plant-based options—without inflammatory responses—should be easy. With your new focus on sustaining good habits, preventing illness, and attending to self-care, most of those eliminated inflammatory foods have lost their luster. Good riddance!

As you enter this phase, I hope you will enjoy more variety on your plate and continue to make decisions that are aligned with your whole-body health goals. But if that doesn't always happen, remember the 10 percent and try not to feel guilty. Making lifelong changes in your routines takes time and patience. You are adding in healthy practices and dropping unhealthy ones. For example, you may need to devote an hour every Sunday to doing meal prep, which may not always be fun, but you can crank up some music or invite a friend to join you. In considering self-care, you may need to unfollow certain people on social media because their messaging is too negative.

DO I NEED TO STAY IN RESET?

Some of my clients prefer to stay in Reset a little longer. They are feeling lighter, healthier, and more in tune. I believe the number one reason clients want to stick with the fundamentals of Reset is that they are excited by seeing the results they had hoped for. Staying in Reset is your prerogative, but do it because you feel as though a couple more weeks could sharpen your new skills, reinforce those better habits, and seal that foundation in cement.

If you are contemplating staying with the Reset phase a little longer, I suggest modifying here and there with some plant-based protein as an addition to your meals. Try lentils first, especially red lentils, which fall apart when cooked and are therefore one of the better digested lentils. Red lentils are also a wonderful addition to soup (see Ginger Pumpkin Soup from Reset). Add a handful of chickpeas here and there in a simple salad. Also, try the Chia Pudding, as this is a delicious and creative way to reap the benefits of that superfood. See how that goes and build on what makes you feel your best, all while considering diversity and optimal sources of nutrition.

If you aren't sure about moving into Maintenance, consider the following to improve upon digestive processes and confidently wipe out those old habits:

- If you are anxious about running out for a burger and fries, consider staying in Reset for another week. While there is nothing wrong with indulging, remember what inflammatory foods can do. Since you are so clean, the combination of oil in the fries, gluten in the bun, and potentially questionable meat sources will most likely have you feeling under the weather. Ask yourself if you feel as though you have quenched the need for any of the inflammatory foods (Foods to Avoid in chapter 2) you set out to cut down on. If this want is a celebratory craving, go for it, but think about sourcing a grass-fed burger, maybe sans the bun for now, and order up a baked potato instead of fries. The latter scenario builds better habits.
- Perhaps you would like to indulge in an ice cream cone. By

all means, buy ice cream if you want it, but become that confident label reader who looks for brands with a mission statement to give the consumer the best possible product. If you suspect that dairy caused you discomfort before Reset, proceed with caution and don't overdue the portion size. If loading up on toppings like crushed Oreos and M&M's were your thing and you can't wait to pile up, consider that you may have not fully squashed that sugar monster just yet. Some of us need a week or two more to fully grasp the confidence and ability to walk away from all the inflammatory sugar, additives, and preservatives these treats present.

- You may not feel completely confident with your prepping skills or routines yet, but please don't stress about that. Finding your new groove takes time. If you have made it this far, that dedication will keep you on track and the routine will unfold accordingly. There are days for those easier meals. As your health and outlook improve, opportunities for more elaborate menu ideas and recipes requiring more time will present themselves.

Compromised digestive processes can also hinder the ability to break down certain foods fully. Therefore, if you are incredibly gassy and uncomfortable, more may be going on. Here are some signs that may indicate a need to stay in Reset a week or two more:

You are lacking sufficient stomach acid (see Your Current Gut Environment). If you suspect the possibility after self-testing, consult a specialist. It is possible to build up vital stomach acid organically with the protocols you have followed in the last three weeks. You can try a modified version of Reset and slowly add in some plant-based proteins, continue with more cooked vegetables as opposed to raw, and continue to take the healing slow and steady for optimal digestion. Leafy salad greens and simple salads are always encouraged to aid in keeping the GI tract clean and fueling good bacteria.

You have unwanted bacteria in your small intestine (see Identifying Food Intolerances, Sensitivities, and Allergies). Small-intestine bacteria is often associated with conditions like IBS, SIBO, or IBD. If you are experiencing symptoms such as undigested food in your stools, eczema, cramping, or uncomfortable gas after meals, this may be the case. If you can't find relief from these symptoms, consulting a health-care professional or functional medicine doctor for further testing will lessen the risk of comorbidities and autoimmune disease.

If you had acid reflux prior to Reset and still don't feel relief after the three weeks, you might continue with only noninflammatory options for several more weeks, then reevaluate. Creating a more alkaline balance comes with time and dedication. If the severity of symptoms is still present, please check with a functional medicine doctor or gastroenterologist to rule out more serious conditions.

Keep in mind that feeling gassy is not always an indicator that you need to stay in Reset. For example, if you indulge in a plate of roasted brussels sprouts or add some sautéed cabbage to a stir-fry, feeling gassy is normal. That's because these cruciferous veggies are known to be top gas producers. It's also possible that you may have eaten too large a portion of cruciferous vegetables or eaten too fast, which could create air pockets. Excess gas is not abnormal in these situations.

Think about how you felt as you started Reset and any concerning issues such as bloating, achy joints, acne, or constipation. Now ask yourself, *How much have these issues improved?* If there has been no relief, and depending on the severity of these symptoms, getting in touch with a medical professional to assess the situation further is your next step.

WHAT IF I MESS UP?

Now that you have established a structured foundation, everything becomes second nature, correct?

Unfortunately, there is no perfect world. Remember that one of the take-home messages with the three-week Reset was that life is not and will never be perfect. We should think of our new selves as works in progress. Catching those curveballs and dealing with life in general puts more than enough on our plates, but we have adopted a more structured, calm, and healthful attitude. We can deal with these situations differently now and do our best to keep on track in every aspect of homeostasis.

While dining out, there may be a flourless chocolate cake in your future. It's okay to celebrate by sharing a slice with a friend or significant other. Savor every morsel with the realization that your efforts have paid off. When you break something as serious as a sugar habit, that accomplishment is a victory you will be very proud of celebrating. In my world, food is meant to bring people together for joyful reasons. Never attach ill thoughts to indulging in something that brings a smile to your face.

And if you do happen to eat the whole slice, please try not to regard this as a weakness. These moments are part of enjoying life. If you ate half a cake, I'd say you might have hit a bump in the road. And that's okay too. Any sort of "messing up" is a learning experience. Consider that you may need some minor repairs to the foundation to strengthen the infrastructure once again. Optimistic attitudes contribute to overall improved health.

If getting back on track after a road bump doesn't pan out, and you feel as though your best intentions flew out the window, you might consider another Reset. If you fall off the horse, get back on. There is no shame, no blaming or waiting for help. Returning to Reset is not admitting defeat, it is just a way to strengthen your foundation and reactivate. This is all you, so get back up, learn from the experience, and ride off into the sunset knowing you've got this.

REINTRODUCING FOODS

Any elimination protocol should be short term. Further healing means reintroducing certain foods to rule out potential sensitivities, though processed and packaged foods are convenience items that should always be kept at a minimum. Digesting properly circles back to efficient body functions, food diversity, and the intake of all essential nutrients, so reintroducing plant-based proteins like beans, nuts, or pure fermented soy products is encouraged. These foods provide the essential nutrients our bodies need to thrive, and we shouldn't exclude them for too long unless an allergy is suspected (see Identifying Food Intolerances, Sensitivities, and Allergies).

Ready to diversify what's on your plate? If so, I will walk you through how to do this with care. This is not something you want to rush through. I repeat, please do not rush the Maintenance phase!

To begin Maintenance, I keep with the whole-food theme to promote more awareness to the benefits of plant-based options. After feeling so much better in Reset, most of my clients are perfectly fine to stick with robust servings of fruits and vegetables. But they're also eager to reintroduce more options like nuts, seeds, and beans. So I've included many delicious plant-based, gluten-free, and dairy-free recipes specifically designed for Maintenance. Your gut is (hopefully) now healthy enough to properly absorb and distribute nutrients without irritation or an imbalance of harmful bacteria. Even so, your gut is not ironclad; adding in foods known to be inflammatory on a regular basis can lead to digestive problems again. So eat mindfully, that is, pay attention to what and how much you're eating so you can identify the culprit.

You are a clean machine. Keep it that way. Here are the most important points to remember when transitioning into Maintenance:

Add in one food group at a time from the eliminated list. Pinpointing potential negative responses is more effective with this method.

Start with lentils. If you're ready to reap the benefits of plant-based protein, fiber, and iron sources, lentils are the place to start. Start with one of the easiest to digest varieties (see French Green Lentil Salad) and pay attention to how your body reacts; if all is well, you can work up to other legumes. Black Bean Soup is another optimal source of plant-based protein, fiber, and many other nutrients. This soup is perfect for transitioning into Maintenance.

Add in some nuts or nut butters as a snack. For me, adding nuts and seeds back into my rotation was an eye-opener. As a chef, experimenting with nuts and adding them whenever I could always made sense. I made nut-based yogurts, spreads, and sauces constantly. After Reset, I realized that my old ways were too much of a burden on my digestive system. That and I was taking in an overabundance of nuts, eating so much because I wasn't absorbing nutrients properly. My body was starving for nutrients, and that shut-off switch was often broken. After Reset, the desire was gone. I still love almond butter with a banana or on a rice cake occasionally, but the craving shifted and, in some ways, vanished. I am more satisfied and satiated and don't pick at snack foods like I used to. I also found that cashews were no longer appealing, and I used to eat them daily. Strange but true!

Cook your veggies, at least at first. Cruciferous vegetables such as broccoli, cabbage, and cauliflower are not inflammatory foods but are harder on the digestive tract for some, especially when raw. But don't avoid these veggies, as they are excellent sources of sulfur, which helps synthesize glutathione, a powerful antioxidant that helps protect your cells from damage. I'll get into oxidative stress more in Issues That May Need Extra Support but protecting your cells from the damaging effects of food is key. To avoid gas with cruciferous vegetables, try eating smaller amounts and more cooked than raw as you ease yourself back into the benefits they offer. When you are feeling more confident, try the Shaved Brussels Sprout Salad with Lemon-Shallot Vinaigrette.

Add animal protein or fish to your meal lineup if you wish. Consider these protein sources in moderation, and buy wild-caught fish and grass-fed meats whenever possible. When animals are raised in their natural environments, they are not prone to disease and illness and are not pumped up with antibiotics.

Drink coffee or tea with food in your stomach. Drinking a beverage with caffeine on an empty stomach can irritate or damage the lining of your gut. It also opens the door for heartburn and unnecessary anxiety. Anxiety gets the cortisol pumping in situations when it's not necessary. If you prefer to stay away from caffeine entirely, run with it.

Limit processed and refined flours if you can. Remember that those simple carbohydrates are the biggest disruptors of the endocrine system. If you don't feel well after having refined bread, pasta, or crackers, you may want to cut them out more often.

Try grain-free versions of your favorite snacks, such as tortillas, chips, and crackers, but remember that even these are convenience items, and it's important to use those label reading skills. For example, corn is an inexpensive crop, the shelf life is long, and its uses in our modern world are abundant. Eighty percent of processed foods contain some sort of byproduct from corn, soy, or wheat. Long-term exposure to synthetic pesticides sprayed on these crops are linked to chronic health conditions and the risk of cognitive impairments and disease.

Kick the sugar habit to the curb, for sure. Processed and artificial sugars are silent killers, and there is no need for them in our lives.

Make this elimination permanent. Find healthier ways to enjoy sweets. See Oatmeal Raisin Cookies.

Avoid packaged and processed items. I know I've said this before, but with inflammatory oils, added sugars, sodium, artificial colorings, additives, and preservatives, these foods are better left on the shelf.

Notice new aversions. It may surprise you that certain foods are no longer appealing. When an inflammatory food becomes unattractive, you have cleared a considerable hurdle. Congratulations! Your body is simply becoming more in tune with what it wants and doesn't. This happens often, particularly with alcohol. The appeal loses its luster because waking up with a clear head takes precedence! Some clients also stay away from eggs because they do not find them appetizing anymore. Listen to and trust your body.

As you navigate Maintenance and add in some eliminated foods, you may react negatively with stomach pains and excessive gas (see Identifying Food Intolerances, Sensitivities, and Allergies). For example, suppose you decide to make one of several delicious salads in the Maintenance section that include beans. Afterward, you feel gassy. This is normal because beans contain gas-producing natural sugars (raffinose and oligosaccharides). Depending on the severity, you may want to eat a smaller portion or try an easier-to-digest bean (such as lentils). Keep in mind that beans are nutrient dense, protein rich, and a great source of fiber. Ease into legumes and beans, as this food source, full of soluble fiber, can boost metabolism and support gut health. What wouldn't be considered normal is if you woke up the next day after an eliminated food with a skin rash, loose stools, or undigested food in your bowel movements. Symptoms like those mentioned could indicate a food sensitivity. Persistent symptoms like these should be discussed with a medical professional.

Be mindful of those eliminated inflammatory foods and how you feel when you have them again. For example, if you add back in a glass of wine every other day and you're suddenly not feeling as good as you did while in Reset, it's time to reevaluate that inflammatory trigger, which could be sugar, nitrates, or gluten. Don't let yourself get back into that uncomfortable place.

With all the scientific information about the benefits of a plant-based shift under your belt, you are equipped to make better choices focused on less inflammation in your body. Reintroducing known inflammatory foods should be done with the mentality that you will either feed the disease or fight it. Also, remember the handy symptoms and food tracker chart (find it in the back of the book). This is a useful tool for charting foods and potential symptoms. Make the better choice more often. That is your new mantra.

INTUITIVE EATING

Intuitive eating is the philosophy that *you* are the expert on your body and its hunger signals. The ideology requires that you make peace with all types of food and listen to what your body tells you is right for you. How refreshing!

To eat intuitively, you must trust your body and your own felt sense of what's "right," which is unique to and deeply rooted in you. The practice also encourages one to honor hunger and challenge the food police. Unfortunately, this does not come about easily for most. There are unreasonable rules in our heads, created and conditioned by years of dieting and the diet culture. Hence, we lose our core values, scrutinize every action, and keep our body and food choices in a constant battle.

The concept of intuitive eating pulls away from the dieting mindset. Healing your relationship with food is a prominent outcome of both the principals of intuitive eating and the Reset program—but it can take time physically and emotionally. If you are holding on to any kind of restrictive ideas about food, diet beliefs, or ill relationships with food, intuitive eating will fail you. Consciously separating physical from emotional hunger creates long-term healthier habits. That said, sitting down to eat and truly enjoying your food without too many interruptions or negative judgments is crucial. You want to be calm, grateful, and appreciative of the food at mealtime, knowing that you are truly nourishing yourself for better wellness. From a health standpoint, these positive actions and emotions are genuinely beneficial for higher levels of self-esteem and better body image. With the progression of more intuitive eating, you'll be less preoccupied with food and lower your risk of emotional eating disorders.

Most clients come to me with the desire to lose weight. They've tried countless diets and are frustrated when unsuccessful attempts leave them guilty and shameful in a culture that praises thinness. When I teach them the fundamentals of intuitive eating practices, they begin to focus on how they feel rather than how they look. This shift in core values is crucial, and means they start to prioritize maintaining whole, nutritious, and gut-friendly choices that are *intuitive*.

Only you can know your body's true needs. Obsessing about losing weight and judging your own food choices inhibit your ability to listen to your body. Intuitive eating opens the lines of communication. Lifestyle modifications take time, so don't be discouraged if it takes a few more weeks to ditch that diet mentality, be at peace, and feel better aligned with the concepts of intuitive eating practices.

PROGRESS, NOT PERFECTION

Positive results you can see and feel are starting to unfold. This is the reward for making change and taking specific steps toward optimal digestive health. The Reset 90/10 program helps your body become more alkaline and less toxic (acidic). Foods you eliminated may have been causing negative responses in your body, so be aware of how you feel when you have them again. A negative reaction may not happen right away, but you will know if something is not agreeing with you. A headache, next-day fogginess, a rash, or extreme gas are examples.

Please don't view these discomforts as setbacks or as evidence that you're doing something "wrong." In fact, take the time to acknowledge how better in tune you are with your body—more so than before you started this program. You have the know-how to get your gut back on track. This awareness is where your progress comes from. You are learning what is best for your body while sometimes splurging for the simple reason of enjoyment without guilt and shaming. In this journey we recognize that there is not one answer or cure-all. For each of us there are so many layers and variables, so as we dig deeper, the work pays off. The overall balance of both worlds is where you find harmony.

IDENTIFYING FOOD INTOLERANCES, SENSITIVITIES, AND ALLERGIES

You have been so clean for the last couple of weeks that it will likely be easier for you to be in tune with your body. Maintenance is the perfect time to assess whether your body has a food sensitivity, intolerance, or allergy—and to respond accordingly to keep your digestive tract healthy. Many of us live with chronic, toxic, or prolonged inflammatory responses for so long that we either tolerate them, ignore them, deem them "normal," or attribute them to another confusing diagnosis. Your recalibrated body will do a good job telling you when it doesn't like something. Pay attention to the signals your body gives you, because you don't want to discredit all the quality time that you have invested in reducing inflammation.

Remember, limiting the uptake of potential antigens (the inflammatory foods you eliminated in Reset) gives the small intestine a break. It provides the opportunity for your body's natural defenses to kick in and build up antibodies. These antibodies play a key role in the immune system and are produced in response to foreign substances like bacteria and viral cells. Antibodies are also created to acknowledge the potential threat of foods, dust, dander, and pollen. With proper healing and without the overabundance of harmful bacteria ruling the environment, not everything entering your gut will be perceived as an invader. Ultimately, our cells, small intestine, and immune responses are strong enough to break down any foreign substance and remove it organically.[75]

Anything extreme in the way of intense cramping, gas shortly after a meal, or runny stools the following day (potential immune responses) may be indicators of a food sensitivity. This doesn't mean that you are allergic to the food, just that you are highly sensitive to it. Immune responses, like allergies, are immediate reactions to foods that should most likely be eliminated from your diet. If you suspect an intolerance or sensitivity, you could consider eliminating this food for a more extended period to further alleviate inflammation to your gut lining. A medical analysis should always be considered to better assess a situation that you feel is out of your control.

Because some reactions associated with a sensitivity can take up to seventy-two hours to appear after reintroducing an offending food, journaling, using a food tracker app, or using the symptoms and food tracker chart at the back of this book can help. Be aware that reintroducing one food group at a time, separated by at least three days, is the best way to effectively pinpoint a potential sensitivity or allergy. So as much as you may want to try some avocado sourdough toast with feta cheese, remember that both bread and cheese could cause adverse reactions, and if you eat them together, you won't know which one is the culprit. Once you're in the clear, that is, showing no signs of inflammation or allergy, you can combine them in meals.

Food intolerances, sensitivities, and allergies each produce different responses in your body. All three categories can have similar symptoms, which can become confusing; however, becoming more in tune with your body and the signals it's giving you can go a long way toward being able to accurately identify the type of reaction you're having. Listening to your immune responses helps you stay healthy for the long term. Let's look more closely at all three of these.

INTOLERANCES

Intolerance is a nonimmune inflammatory response from your body not being able to break down certain foods. Without vital stomach acid or digestive enzymes, which our bodies should make naturally, we develop food intolerances. Schools of thought state that long-term meds, stress, and an overly acidic environment can also contribute to a decrease in stomach acid and digestive enzymes, resulting in a food intolerance. A runny nose, nausea, gas, cramping, or diarrhea are typical reactions to food intolerance. The most common food intolerances are lactose, a sugar found in cow's milk; casein, a protein found in milk; and gluten, a protein present in grains such as wheat, barley, and rye. For reference, lactose in sheep's and goat's milk is not as prevalent but still exists. Casein is also a protein in goat's and sheep's milk, but in a different form, making those options more tolerable for some.

Food intolerances do *not* trigger immune reactions. So, while a food intolerance is *not* life-threatening, if one continues to ignore the signs, the problem will only get worse. Let's use dairy as an example. If you suspect lactose intolerance, you could be deficient in the enzyme lactase. Lactase is needed to break down lactose, the sugar found

in cow's milk. If left untreated, more severe digestive issues can present. The most common symptoms of lactose intolerance are nausea,
bloating, and gas pains in the stomach and chest area after consuming
dairy products.

If you suspect an intolerance but have cut out dairy products like
milk, cheese, and yogurt, read labels for the not-so-obvious dairy
pseudonyms sneaking into foods, such as whey, curds, buttermilk,
cream, and milk powder.

In Maintenance, if you suspect a food intolerance, limit the offending food *and* limit the amount of other inflammatory foods you reintroduce. For example, if you suspect lactose intolerance, keep dairy
out for a couple more weeks. But also limit processed foods and go
back to Foods to Avoid in the second chapter. Allow your body to continue detoxing organs and building up more vital stomach acid (see
Adequate Stomach Acid) and support optimal digestion with plant-
based foods high in digestive enzymes (see Digestive Enzymes). You
are literally giving your body more TLC and fine-tuning that best-case
scenario for you.

If you want to be sure you have a lactose intolerance, consider con-
firming with a hydrogen breath test or lactose intolerance test. You
can also work with a specialist who can guide you with enzyme or
quality probiotic supplementation. You might exclude dairy products
altogether and try reintroducing them in several weeks. Another theory suggests that we may be able to train our body to produce lactase by consuming small quantities daily.[76] Bottom line: your body is
unique, and you should do what you feel most comfortable with.

SENSITIVITIES

Food sensitivity (also referred to as delayed food allergy) occurs when
our immune system is reactive to a particular food or food additive,
resulting in the release of specific immunoglobulin G (IgG) antibodies. Antibodies are protein components produced by immune cells to
neutralize toxins. The IgG antibody is the most abundant immunoglobulin present in most tissues and blood. The function of an IgG antibody is to recognize, remember, and block an antigen (food, bacteria,
virus, or other microorganism recognized as a threat). The backlash of

these repeated threats—and antibodies trying to fight off the perceived enemy—could include symptoms such as headaches, acid reflux, fatigue, joint pain, bloating, constipation, diarrhea, and brain fog.[77] The conditions associated with food sensitivities are migraines, Crohn's, depression, weight gain, eczema, ear infections, colitis, IBS, and asthma.

Chronic stress, in addition to frequent antibiotic use, NSAIDs, and excessive amounts of soda, coffee, alcohol, and sugar also play a significant part in the development of food sensitivities. This is another example of oxidative stress in the body. Over time, these actions and choices significantly break down cells and disrupt the precious mucosal lining and permeability of the gut. This breakdown means there are microscopic holes in the lining of your small intestine that allow food particles, toxins, and bacteria to escape into the bloodstream. This is a heavy burden on the immune system. The thinning of the gut lining is referred to as a mucosal immunoglobulin A (IgA) antibody response. IgA secretion is our first line of defense against viral and bacterial infection. This antibody wants to help us fight off sickness, but the constant release of these IgA antibodies potentially opens the door to conditions like leaky gut syndrome.[78] Our mucosal lining cushions and protects our cells, traps pathogens, and protects cells from external toxins. A damaged lining can cause leaky gut, which is associated with the breakdown of immune health and the body mistakenly making antibodies against healthy tissue.

As with an IgG response, the antibodies dwindle and the body grows weaker from constantly fighting off perceived threats. For most experiencing chronic pain, their immune systems have become too weak from fighting the symptoms for a prolonged period.[79] There is no general in this army giving instruction, there are just fighters struggling to keep you healthy. You need to guide this army of defenders with less inflammation and stress. When we heal the gut lining, we support immune functions and can get a better grip on autoimmune disease associated with inflammation.

The good news is that pinpointing a food sensitivity and removing the threat typically results in a noticeable improvement of symptoms. Further modifications like adopting more plant-based options, cutting out processed foods, and even keeping animal protein to a minimum can significantly improve irritating ailments. Moving away from the standard American diet is a pivotal first step in maintaining remission and finding relief from something like Crohn's disease or IBS.[80]

Gaining clarity on deeper issues may require medical testing with the aid of an integrative or functional medicine doctor. Our immune system is designed to protect us. Still, autoimmune diseases, chronic illness, and excess inflammation can lead to elevated antibodies concentrating on one organ, such as the thyroid. When excess inflammation spirals out of control, conditions like Hashimoto's and Graves' result from high antibodies in the thyroid. They may require working with a practitioner who can evaluate your adrenal glands, thyroid, and hormones through more comprehensive testing.[81]

As with intolerances, dairy and gluten seem to be the most prevalent sensitivities. Some of us are better off keeping gluten completely out of our diets. Gluten appears to be a trigger for many and is high on the list of IgG immune responses to food. More research also proposes glyphosate, the active ingredient in the herbicide Roundup, is a major contributor to the uptick of celiac and gluten sensitivities worldwide.[82] If you suspect a gluten sensitivity, consider testing from a gastroenterologist or functional medicine specialist to rule out celiac disease. After the three-week elimination, you will make pinpointing intolerances and sensitivities so much easier if you follow the one-food-at-a-time reintroduction protocol. Food elimination appears to be the most successful for healing gut permeability, but to fully restore and rebuild, time and commitment are essential. As these conditions did not happen overnight, practice patience, knowing the rewards of health are preferred over illness.

If further evaluation is what you seek, look to a specialist for an IgG test (Genova and Great Plains have reputable results). The most frequent food specific IgG antibodies identified (highest to lowest) are kola nuts (flavoring agent in soda, popular energy drinks, and performance enhancers), brewer's yeast (bread, beer, wine, and alcohol), gluten products (wheat, barley, rye, spelt, and wheat starch), red kidney beans, corn, and eggs. An IgA test can also help; it measures blood levels of IgA in the stomach's mucous membrane layer.

In addition, be mindful of rest and digest, stress, and other healthful adjustments you have been building on to remove internal inflammation. When we give our bodies these supportive means, our immune reactive antibodies become more robust and better equipped to defend against real foreign invaders like bacteria, viruses, and environmental exposure. The bottom line is that the best tool for identifying potential sensitivities is prudent observation and trial and error. During Reset, you have removed the inflammatory foods associated with these uncomfortable and bothersome sensitivities, and you have also started the healing process your immune system thrives on. With this foundation, sensitivities can be reduced or eradicated.

ALLERGIES

An allergic reaction is an instantaneous immune immunoglobulin E (IgE) response to an antigen that has entered the body. The reaction produces hypersensitive inflammatory symptoms like hives, vomiting, lip swelling, itching, trouble swallowing, and breathing issues associated with the release of histamines. Common food allergens include soybeans, wheat, shellfish, fish, peanuts, cow's milk, eggs, and tree nuts.

Can you develop an allergy? Is it possible to grow out of an allergy? Can you be tested for specific allergens? The answer is yes to all three.

For example, let's say you eat some cheese and instantaneously develop hives on your arms. Here's what's going on in your body. Seeing the cheese as a foreign toxin, your white blood cells react by producing chemicals and IgE antibodies to bind to the protein in the cheese. On cue from the immune system, the release of histamines—formed to protect and get those allergens out of your body—brings about inflammation and itching in the form of hives. IgE related food allergies generally do not go away, and it is commonly advisable to stay away from trigger foods, but an allergy can decrease over time if an individual's health progresses. The improvement of overall gut health contributes to the strength of the immune system.

If you suspect allergies, sensitivities, or intolerances to food or additives, preservatives, or dyes, I encourage you to become proactive by having annual antibody testing. The expertise of an integrative doctor provides more comprehensive testing and the ability to dig deeper for a root cause if dietary changes don't get you to where you want to be. There are immunoglobin blood panels specifically designed to test foods, dyes, inhalants, and mold to name a few. You might also consider consulting a naturopath. Most naturopaths look for root causes before considering medications that just treat symptoms. With leaky gut, IBS, malnutrition, and other issues, utilizing supplements can be essential for some.[83]

Checking in with the right professional may initially come with some out-of-pocket expenses, but compare that to what chronic illnesses, autoimmune diseases, comorbidities, and other debilitating diseases will do to your bank account. An ounce of prevention and proactive measures will take you far.

BECOMING A CONFIDENT LABEL READER

If you are serious about becoming more aware of additives and potentially harmful ingredients in your food choices, embrace the research and scrutinize labels. We all wonder why autoimmune and chronic illnesses dominate our world today, with scientific research reporting that in the last two decades, there has been a significant increase in food allergies, asthma, autism spectrum disorder, and fibromyalgia.[84] But the truth is right on the label, and our bodies pay the price. Reading through labels doesn't have to become your new full-time job, but trust that it will become easier if you master the 101 on ingredients.

CITRIC ACID

Citric acid is used to stabilize, preserve, and disinfect against viruses and bacteria in packaged foods. In the late 1700s, we produced citric acid solely from lemon juice. In the early 1900s, researchers discovered that synthetic citric acid could also be manufactured from the black mold *Aspergillus niger*. This fabricated formation differs vastly from what's found naturally in citrus fruits. It is also a known allergen, yet 99 percent of the world's production of manufactured citric acid is formulated this way.[85]

Manufactured citric acid is cheap and easy to mass produce. It boosts acidity, enhances flavor, and preserves the ingredients. While that may be great for shelf life, it is wreaking havoc inside your body. It can be found in cleaning agents, nutritional supplements, and endless packaged foods such as sodas, energy drinks, juices, candies, frozen foods, canned and jarred foods, instant oatmeal, powdered beverages, some dairy, the list goes on and on.

There are many types of black mold, and the most common health risks associated with exposure are respiratory issues, coughing, sneezing, eye irritation, rashes, fatigue, and headaches. Inflammation at its best. Hmm, no thanks.

SUGAR SUBSTITUTES

Artificial and processed sugar both bring about trouble. There is much controversy around whether the FDA studies that deem sugar substitutes, artificial sweeteners, and sugar alcohols safe are accurate. If they are free from danger, why do these findings also suggest that it's best to limit them?[86] Even more, why then are these intense sweeteners comparatively as addictive as cocaine?[87]

Some artificial sweeteners or sugar substitutes are derived from sugar alcohols. These include zero-calorie sweeteners like mannitol, erythritol, isomalt, and sorbitol. They can trick the brain into promoting more sugar cravings and a false sense of hunger while interfering with insulin balance.

Other sugar substitutes are marketed as "natural sweeteners" because they are made from real sugar. Remember, even table sugar is highly processed. These "natural" low calorie sweeteners include sucralose (Splenda), saccharin (Sweet'N Low) and aspartame (Equal). While made from real sugar, these sweeteners undergo a chemical process that turns them into a synthetic chemical. Our bodies do not recognize these chemical structures and they often go undigested, passing through our gut and altering beneficial bacteria.

Other sugar substitutes and artificial sweeteners include

- Acesulfame-K
- Advantame
- Agave
- Alitame
- Cyclamate
- Dextrose

- Fructose
- Glucose
- High-fructose corn syrup
- Neotame

Sugar substitutes bring about inflammation and the onset of excess abdominal weight. When consumed regularly, the compounds raise blood sugar and insulin levels. More and more research shows that a typical response is increased blood sugar levels that take longer to show up than with a teaspoon of natural sugar, meaning the ill effects are slow moving. When foods made with artificial sweeteners are consumed, these bogus ingredients' metabolic disturbances will trigger and manipulate negative pleasure responses in the brain, causing cravings for more calories in the form of sugar. If this is an addictive response, long-term effects can include a host of alarming neurological issues such as unstable moods, loss of memory, and dementia.[88]

Artificial sweeteners are so ubiquitous that you can find them in nonfood items around your home. They turn up in the electrolyte drinks we give our kids when they are ill, chewing gum, laxatives, mouthwash, and toothpaste. Yoplait yogurt proudly states there is no aspartame in their products, yet sucralose and acesulfame potassium show up on the ingredients list. Please do not jump on that "sugar-free" bandwagon. It's headed right into a world full of cognitive, digestive, blood sugar, and addiction issues you do not want.

GLUTEN-FREE

Just because something is labeled "gluten-free" doesn't mean that it's better for you.

The GF trend has led many manufacturers to come up with marketing scams to make money on what's popular. And people are eagerly loading up on these products that offer no nutritional value. If a product is packaged as gluten-free, the FDA states that less than twenty parts per million of the food will contain a byproduct of wheat. But if you have been diagnosed with celiac, consuming even just a little gluten could be detrimental to your health. More-specific third-party certifications such as certified gluten-free ensure a higher standard for those that need or want products without the potential adversities.

When purchasing gluten-free products, look for whole grains like chickpea, quinoa, teff, or buckwheat flour listed first on the ingredient label. Brown rice flour is better if it is organic. Avoid excessive fillers and starches such as tapioca, potato, and corn, as these are frequently added to these convenience foods and will cause blood sugar spikes and only provide empty calories. The same mindfulness applies to excess omega-6 inflammatory oils (canola, cottonseed, soybean, vegetable), refined sugars, and xanthan gum, which should be ingested in moderation, especially if you suspect gastrointestinal issues.

THE 5/20 RULE

When picking better products at the market, abiding by the 5/20 rule can help. The 5/20 rule references the daily value (DV) percentages on a nutrition facts label. It reminds us that, according to guidelines from the FDA, 5 percent DV or less of a nutrient per serving is considered low and 20 percent DV or more of a nutrient per serving is considered high.

So how do you use this ranking to your advantage? When reaching for an item on the shelf, check its nutrition label. In general, if it's low (5 percent or less) in things like trans fats, sodium, cholesterol, and added sugars, and high (20 percent or more) in good nutrients like vitamins, minerals, fiber, and protein, that food item is a keeper.

But as I've reiterated throughout this book, each of us has unique dietary needs that also shift over time. So consider specific categories and how they pertain to your needs or restrictions, such as with your sodium, fiber, protein, and fat intake. Evaluate and adjust as needed.

STOCKING YOUR PANTRY

Clients always ask me what I recommend when it comes to products. They want to know what brands I like, what I always keep stocked in my pantry, and of course, my kitchen shortcuts on the days when I need something quick and easy. Please keep in mind that these are mostly convenience foods. We all need a little assistance at times—just remember that sourcing intact fruits and vegetables whenever possible will help you feel your best.

Many of the brands and ingredients I use are gluten-free and organic. Nonorganic products, particularly rice and oats, have the potential to contain an abundance of pesticides, which maximizes your exposure to harmful chemicals. Oats, unless stated "certified gluten-free," can become problematic if you have celiac or gluten sensitivities. Over time, using nonorganic products compromises your digestive tract.

When you find a good product you can trust, be creative, reinvent the typical meal, and have fun experimenting. Gaining confidence in the kitchen will have you turning out delicious, nutritious, and satisfying meals in no time.

PANTRY MUST-HAVES

Almond butter: Woodstock and 365. Almonds should be the only ingredient with no added sugar or oil. If your supermarket makes freshly ground nut butters, there's nothing better.

Brown rice cakes: Lundberg and Trader Joe's. Add some hummus, an avocado or guacamole (savory), or try refried beans and a little guacamole or salsa (salty). Sometimes a teaspoon of almond butter and banana slices (sweet) does the trick. Be creative when you need a quick snack!

Canned pumpkin, butternut squash, and sweet potatoes: 365, Brad's Organic, and Farmer's Market. When you are stocked and ready to go, make something like the Sweet Potato Muffins or Roasted Vegetables and Mushroom Stew.

Chia seeds: 365, Navitas Organics, and Spectrum. White or black chia seeds work in Chia Pudding and Very Berry Chia Oats. Black chia seeds provide slightly more protein and white have more omega-3s.

Dried fruit: Woodstock has good-quality dried fruit options. Look for brands with no added sugars. For dried Smyrna figs, look online for Sunny Fruit.

Dried mulberries: Typically these can be found in specialty stores near the raisins. You can order Anthony's Goods online. Oven-Dried Mulberries is the "new" nutrient-dense granola.

Frozen vegetables: 365 has a variety and Cascadian Farm's pre-riced broccoli, sweet potato, and cauliflower are super convenient for Roasted Sweet Potato Fried Rice.

Hearts of palm linguini and pasta sheets: Natural Heaven offers great pasta substitutes you can use to build fresh, cold salad-type dishes. Look for other brands with only hearts of palm on the ingredients list and avoid brands with citric acid.

Kale chips: Make your own at home, but if you do buy them, watch out for inflammatory oils (corn, soy, vegetable, safflower) or eat them in moderation.

Ketchup: Primal Kitchen is the only brand that I have found to have no added sugars. Red Duck, Trader Joe's, and Annie's come close but do contain a small amount of added sugars. Please do not buy ketchup with high-fructose corn syrup.

Lentils and beans: 365 and Eden are great sources of plant-based protein and fiber. Most supermarkets carry their own organic brand. Look for canned versions that are BPA-free and/or organic. If you are cooking dried beans, look for sprouted types also. Soaking dried beans before cooking is always recommended (see Pressure Cooker Beans).

Oats: For GF rolled oats, which is what I use for overnight oats and oatmeal cookies, use Bob's Red Mill, One Degree Organic Foods, and 365. For steel cut oats, use any organic GF brand.

Pecan and Medjool date rolls: Natural Delights. Typically found in most stores in the dried fruit area near the produce. They also make date and coconut rolls that are a perfect snack!

Pink Himalayan salt: This is my go-to as it has less sodium than regular table salt. The pink salt also has trace minerals of iron, manganese, zinc, and calcium.

Plant-based milks: Malk, Elmhurst 1925, Three Trees, and Willa's Kitchen. Look for brands that do not contain the following additives as they are known to cause gas and bloating: guar gum, carrageenan, added sugars, sunflower oil, gellan gum, and sunflower lecithin.

Plant-based yogurts: Harmless Harvest, Forager Project, Nancy's, and Lavva—so yummy layered on Chia Pudding and Very Berry Chia Oats.

Rice: Lotus Foods (pink, jade pearl, and black forbidden rice), any sprouted rice, brown rice, wild rice.

Rice noodles: Lotus Foods, Explore Cuisine.

Sea seasonings: Maine Coast Sea Seasonings (Triple Blend Flakes,

Kelp Granules, and Dulse with Garlic). These are an excellent source of vitamins, minerals, and iodine. Do not take any iodine supplementation if you are on thyroid medication, as supplements can interfere with absorption issues you may already have.

Seaweed snacks: SeaSnax. So yummy and a great source of sea vegetables or try making them at home (see Baked Seaweed Snacks).

Spices: Frontier Co-Op, Mrs. Dash Garlic and Herb, and 365.

Vegetable stocks and broths: 365 and Trader Joe's. Most stores carry their own organic brands. Many conventical brands contain high-fructose corn syrup and preservatives, so always read the label.

Tahini: Roland and Artisana Organics. Many of the salad dressings and sauces in my recipes use tahini. Tahini has great minerals such as copper and zinc—which are essential for optimal thyroid function and hormone production—and iron, and is a rich source of B vitamins, vital omega fats, magnesium, and calcium.

PANTRY NICE-TO-HAVES

Almond flour, chickpea flour, or coconut flour tortillas: Siete Family Foods. These offer a great and tasty alternative to gluten and corn products. Keep them in your freezer and turn leftover broccoli rabe and a can of refried beans into a tasty and enjoyable quesadilla.

Bean soup mix: Frontier has a lot of soup mixes—so great for a quick soup or stew-like meal. I use them as a base and add in extra frozen vegetables and a handful of cooked pasta, rice, or quinoa at the end. Great for meals and leftovers in a pinch (see Doctored-Up Bean Soup Mixes).

Precooked beets: Love Beets and Auga. If you love beets, these are low in calories and high in valuable vitamins and minerals and are typically found in the produce aisle. Perfect for What a Veggie Burger!

Breakfast cereals: Three Wishes, Lovebird Foods, Forager Project, 365, Nature's Path, and One Degree Organic Foods.

Brown rice quinoa pasta: 365 and Trader Joe's. Add some sautéed vegetables, fresh herbs, and vegetable broth for a complete and healthy meal. Making a minestrone soup and adding some cooked pasta to your finished product is also a plus for added nutrients (see Black Lentil Minestrone).

Enchilada sauce: Frontera and Siete both have great premade enchilada sauces to help you out with dinner (see Vegetable Enchiladas). Sometimes I get wild and mix red and green enchilada sauce together.

Fruit powders: Navitas Organics Pomegranate Powder and Navitas Organics Acai Powder (see Chia Pudding and Very Berry Chia Oats).

Gluten-free bread: GluteNull and Simple Kneads. Look for a brand that has close to three or more grams of fiber per serving. A great snack is toasted bread with half a mashed avocado, hummus, a touch of Sun-Dried Tomato Spread, and a sprinkle of dried dulse blend.

Gluten-free pasta: 365, Explore Cuisine, Chickapea, Big Green Organic Food, and Lotus Foods are all great brands of plant-based pastas. King Soba has good-quality buckwheat pastas as well.

Ground hempseed: Bob's Red Mill, Nutiva, and Navitas Organics.

Hemp hearts: Manitoba Harvest, Navitas, Spectrum, and Bob's Red Mill.

Hot sauce: Siete, Red Clay, and Primal Kitchen are all great brands when you're in the mood for a kick of mild or hot spice (see the Zesty Baked Cauliflower Bites).

Pancake and waffle mix: Bob's Red Mill Gluten-Free.

Plant-based protein powders: Naked Seed, Sprout Living, Truvani, Nutiva, and Garden of Life.

Pumpkin, sunflower, and white watermelon seeds: Look for these online: Go Raw and True Elements. These are a great way to add a pop of fiber, healthy fats, vital vitamins, minerals, and antioxidants to a salad, pasta dish, snack, parfait, or muffins. White watermelon seeds are usually found in seedless watermelons and are immature black seeds that pack a punch of nutrients including protein, folate, iron, zinc, magnesium, and potassium.

Refried beans: Amy's and 365 are best. Look for organic, BPA-free canned brands for Quesadillas, Vegetable Enchiladas, and Green Lentil Lasagna with a Mexican twist.

Rice-based tortillas: Food for Life. Look for these in the freezer section.

Salsa: Look for any mild, organic salsa. It's another good item to stock up on (see Vegetable Enchiladas).

Sun-dried tomatoes: Trader Joe's sells sun-dried tomatoes in a small three-ounce bag (see Sun-Dried Tomato Spread).

CHAPTER 12

The Whole-Body Lifestyle

In the last three weeks, you have put out a fire in your gut and cut down the inflammation considerably. Maintenance furthers this journey by strengthening the gut habitat and enhancing cognitive communication. But reaching the Maintenance phase doesn't necessarily mean you're done and that everything will be perfect from here on out. Your health is and always will be a work in progress that requires intention and deliberate action. Just as your gut microbiome is always changing, so too is your life. In this chapter, we'll take a look at how options on and off the plate can support optimal health across mind, body, and spirit.

Take a moment to think about what "healthy" means to you. Consider that health is not just physical, it's a state of mind. It's also unique to each of us and changes over time. As we age, reducing the risk of diseases should be a top priority, but most of us do not consider that subject until we're faced with adversity. I urge you to aim for preventive measures when it comes to your health, instead of treating the problem after it's full blown.

There is a connection between diet and disease, but your chance of improving your health strengthens every time you make a better choice. When that foundation is given consistent TLC, your risks of advanced and full-blown complications lessen. A healthy and hearty immune system clears obstacles effortlessly. Health is about finding balance. Most of us are well aware that the couch-potato mentality is a stable predictor of ill health and an increased risk of cardiovascular disease, obesity, hypertension, and poor mental well-being. But as you think about your whole-body health, keep in mind that too much exercise can backfire, disrupting precious hormonal functions.

The considerations that follow are merely food for thought as you navigate what comes next. The wonderful thing about evolution is that you get to constantly reinvent and update to be the best version of yourself without judgment. When we don't evolve, we become stuck, so take it one day at a time as you figure out what the healthiest version of you looks like. While browsing through the following considerations, consider what works best for you and sidestep what works only for someone else.

MIND

REVIEW PRIMARY AND SECONDARY FOODS

A significant part of health coach training from the Institute for Integrative Nutrition states that when primary food is balanced and satiated, your life feeds you, making what you actually eat secondary.

We have covered many factors that impact well-being. When balance is off in any facet of your life, check in with your primary foods—your relationships, physical health, spirituality, career, and what you do for pleasure—to determine what's missing. For example, if you are feeling hungry, is it because you did not eat a well-balanced lunch? Or could it be that an argument with a partner has thrown you into a tailspin of emotions, leading you to seek comfort, support, and serenity through food? If you are feeling stressed, consider whether you can nourish your body through some heart-pumping exercise, rest, or a spiritual break (a five-minute meditation counts!) rather than a pint of ice cream.

When we are more conscious of triggers to reach for secondary foods—what we actually consume—we are better able to pause and consider whether a focus on primary foods is what we really need. Finding balance among all domains of your life will ultimately contribute to an overall sense of fulfillment, satisfaction, and well-being.

COMMIT TO YOUR NEW MINDSET

It may surprise you to discover that, along with tangible digestive benefits, completing Reset has made you more mindful. That's by design. I created Reset 90/10 to jump-start positive lifestyle changes, starting with the gut. Hopefully you are also seeing benefits from practicing self-care, becoming more attuned to environmental stressors and how to manage them, and noticing and working on imbalances in life domains beyond food. I urge you to keep up the good work!

The gut-brain connection regulates precious hormones such as cortisol, serotonin, dopamine, and melatonin. As a refresher, an adverse gut-brain chemical reaction can create anxiety, inflammation, excess weight, cravings, depression, sleepless nights, and dementia. To keep your microbiome and immune responses strong, check in often with whether you are taking on too much. Reduce chronic stress and anxiety along with excessive exercise. Put your to-do list on hold and do something that makes you happy!

Your new mindset is being shaped by the self-care acts you have been establishing. This improved set of beliefs will influence both your mental and physical reset. As you navigate Maintenance, the goal is to embrace growth and positive change, and this will look different for everyone. Start by asking yourself, *What makes me happy? What keeps me positive? How can I prioritize my self-care?*

For me, happiness comes from following through on my intentions. I personally dislike the statement "I can't," so I have a persistent streak. But then there are the days when I have to say, "No more; I need a break." Those are the times when I prioritize my self-care: I grab my Kindle and escape into a good book.

But what works for me may not work for you. If journaling makes you happy, make that a priority. There are many proven benefits of journaling, from keeping track of intentions, goals, and growth to reducing stress and anxiety. If affirmations keep you positive, incorporate them into your daily routine. The same goes for meditation, visualization, spending time in nature, and regularly making time for important people in your life.

Commit to a growth mindset, which means you are willing to continue to check in with yourself. Listen to your body so you can celebrate when it feels happy and slow down when it gets overwhelmed. You have the tools to make changes before inflammation, chronic fatigue, or burnout take over. Make the mindset work in your favor and find your source of inspiration.

ANTINUTRIENTS

A new buzzword you might have heard is "antinutrients." This refers to compounds that inhibit the body's ability to absorb nutrients. Some theories propose that beans and nightshade vegetables (e.g., tomatoes and peppers) can cause adverse reactions, potentially inhibit the absorption of nutrients, and should be eliminated because they are high in lectins and therefore toxic to our bodies. Active lectins are proteins that bind to carbohydrates causing digestive problems and intestinal permeability.

However, there is very little scientific evidence that supports this. In fact, actively avoiding so many plant-based proteins such as lentils; beans; nuts; grains; seeds; and vegetables like tomatoes, eggplants, and peppers could potentially backfire. In addition to vital vitamins and nutrients, many of these foods contain natural prebiotics and the fiber that feeds healthy gut flora.

Who is eating raw beans or grains? Most lectins are destroyed by soaking, sprouting, and cooking. Refrigeration further eliminates harmful lectins. Research also suggests that the nutritional value of nightshades outweighs the potential toxins from lectins.[89] Rather than worry about lectins, let's aim to eliminate sugary foods, processed food products, and anything with little or no fiber, and increase our intake of antioxidants and essential mineral compounds.

INTERMITTENT FASTING

Intermittent fasting is a diet that varies mealtime schedules to cycle between fasting and eating on a regular schedule. Fasting methods vary but include alternate-day fasting and periodic abstaining. Though this might work for many, these restrictive behaviors, especially for women, are harmful to precious hormones, fertility, and bone health. Fasting can become a stressor for the body. Don't we all deal with enough stress (emotional, physiological, and environmental) regularly?

If you are not sleeping through the night; have thyroid or blood sugar issues; are under much stress; have a history of eating disorders; or typically experience fatigue, mood swings, hunger, reduced energy, or lack of concentration; consider that intermittent fasting may be making matters worse. In addition, restrictive dieting, fasting, and counting can negatively spiral into distorted eating habits. When your body experiences prolonged periods without food, the levels of cortisol—a hormone associated with stress—become elevated. Increased cortisol production over time contributes to many hormonal imbalances. Ignoring our body's biological hunger cues could lead to food obsession, increased hunger, and bingeing.

Healthy habits promote balance both physically and mentally. One's eating habits should leave one energized, calm, and satisfied.

SYMPTOMS YOU SHOULD NOT IGNORE

Having a health scare should prompt a reaction to make changes for the better, yet many of us ignore the signals our bodies send us, mainly because we are too busy and hope they will pass. The following symptoms are warning signs from your body, letting you know something is wrong, so don't ignore them:

- Acid reflux
- Bloating
- Bowel changes
- Chronic fatigue
- Dry skin
- Itching
- Joint pain
- Minimal sleep
- Sudden unexplained pain
- Unintentional weight loss or gain

At times, something like mild acid reflux could result from a spicy meal you aren't used to eating. But persistent and nagging pain that prompts repeated over-the-counter acid blockers will negatively alter your vital stomach acid. In addition, when your esophagus is consistently exposed to stomach acid, more severe reflux (GERD) results. The snowball effect of these untreated and aggravated conditions can lead to ulcers, chest pain, trouble swallowing, Barrett's esophagus, and esophageal cancer. These kinds of serious issues can be prevented and managed.

If you experience sudden, severe, or chronic changes, an evaluation with a health professional is probably a good idea. It's better to find out that your concerning symptom isn't severe than to ignore it until a more dangerous and life-threatening situation arises. Listen to your body, note all symptoms, and share them in detail with a trusted doctor. Time is of the essence; therefore, preventive measures are a life-saving proactive choice.

BODY

YOUR CURRENT GUT ENVIRONMENT

Your current gut environment has improved exceptionally in the last several weeks. You have avoided the pitfalls of processed foods, amped up digestive health with calming foods, and incorporated more alkaline and fiber-rich choices that provide both probiotic and prebiotic benefits. Hopefully, your sugar habits have been kicked, your sleep has improved, your stress is well managed, and your daily self-care routines are enhanced.

Maintaining the correct balance from this point on requires your dedication and diligence to reinforce both physical and mental clarity. In addition, supporting a healthy gut sets the stage for better cognitive health, improved immune functions, and fewer negative stress responses.

ADEQUATE STOMACH ACID

Low stomach acid (or low hydrochloric acid, HCL) triggers poor digestive activity. When food and nutrients do not fully break down, they

Mitochondria

The mitochondria are the life force of cells in our body. Each one of us has unique mitochondrial DNA inherited from our mothers; therefore, siblings from the same mother have similar mitochondrial DNA. The mitochondrion is an essential aspect of our survival. We rely on its essential role in creating energy for proper cellular function. Every biological process depends on converting energy properly. Without normal cell function, we do not perform as we should: we age rapidly and can be affected by heart, brain, muscular, and gastrointestinal complications. Mitochondrial diseases are often long-term, genetically inherited disorders such as poor growth, developmental delays, muscle weakness, fatigue, hearing loss, seizures, strokes, heart failure, diabetes, and kidney failure. Mitochondrial dysfunction, on the other hand, typically happens as we age. Our cells don't work as efficiently and degenerative breakdown begins to occur. If we do not support the immune system, free radicals appear, causing cell oxidation, which can lead to premature aging and a host of diseases.

The force of the mitochondria would safely suggest that their presence is that of a power plant in our body. A body supported by foods high in antioxidants, low stress, and proper exercise can safely interact with free radicals and terminate the chain reaction before vital molecules are damaged. The bottom line is that if the immune system is not regulated, the body has trouble determining which cells are healthy and which aren't. Subsequently, we have inflammation and infection, autoimmune and chronic illness. Untreated and ignored, inflammation will take over. The more support and attention these key players receive, the better the overall outcome.

sit in the stomach too long and cause bacteria to build up. Undigested foods are often the beginning of many chronic health issues—one example is food intolerance. Common causes of low stomach acid include stress, age, vitamin deficiencies (zinc and vitamin B), medications, *H. pylori*, and stomach surgeries. Chronic health conditions linked to low stomach acid are allergies, thyroid issues, acne, lupus, asthma, eczema, osteoporosis, and other autoimmune disorders.

Please take the opportunity to see if any of these symptoms are concerning you at this point:

- Bloating, belching, burning, and excessive gas immediately after meals
- A sense of fullness even with smaller meals
- Bad breath, indigestion, diarrhea, or constipation
- Heartburn
- Weak, peeling, and cracked fingernails
- Dilated blood vessels in the cheeks and nose (rosacea)
- Acne, eczema, and other skin conditions
- Iron deficiency symptoms such as fatigue, paleness, shortness of breath, and dry and damaged hair or skin
- Abdominal pain, diarrhea, gas and bloating, itching around the rectum or vulva, fatigue, and stomach tenderness—symptoms of chronic intestinal parasites and dysbiosis (abnormal gut flora)
- Undigested food in the stool
- Chronic yeast infections
- Chronic anxiety

During the last three weeks, in addition to calming the gut's environment, you have been naturally building up stomach acid by limiting processed foods, properly chewing your food, and becoming mindful of stressful situations (see Too Little Acid for a refresher). But if levels are still low, further treatment with the help of a professional may be necessary. Treatment is dependent on the severity of symptoms. Effective and efficient monitoring would be the best course of action, but remember, prescription and over-the-counter acid blockers will only deplete stomach acid more or raise the acidity levels in that

Self-Testing for Low HCL

You can determine if you need more HCL through a simple home test called the bicarb test. While this may not be the most accurate or scientific method of testing, it is an insightful baseline for those seeking answers. It is important to take the test first thing in the morning and collect data for several days. Try it again in two weeks and save the data. Having this information readily available is so helpful if working with a healthcare professional.

Mix ¼ teaspoon of bicarbonate of soda (baking soda) in about 4 ounces of water and drink on an empty stomach first thing in the morning, before eating or drinking. Set a timer for three minutes. If you have sufficient stomach acid levels, the bicarbonate converts into carbon dioxide gas, which should cause belching in less than three minutes. If belching doesn't happen within three minutes, your stomach acid is low. Note that smaller and repeated belches could result from swallowing air while drinking this solution.

Some clients complain of stomach pain after a meal. If this is you, another at-home test would be to take a tablespoon of straight lemon juice after a meal when pain is present. If the pain goes away, it could be another indicator of low stomach acid. If the pain persists or gets worse, it may possibly be too much acid or the beginning of an ulcer. This may signal the need for a medical professional.

environment too much once you go off the medication. Get to the root cause. Our stomachs need the appropriate balance of acid to break down foods properly.[90]

Digestive changes or concerning symptoms can be addressed and managed by a naturopathic practitioner. The right practitioner can help address, treat, and oversee the underlying cause. For this case, supplements might help. In conjunction with the enzyme pepsin, HCL supplementation (betaine hydrochloride) may help increase the acidity needed in your stomach. These supplements assist in breaking down proteins into the essential amino acids our bodies need to thrive.

DIGESTIVE ENZYMES

As you know, digestive enzymes are needed to break down fats, proteins, and carbohydrates. There are many different points in the digestive process when vital enzymes are released and activated.

Think about food cooking on the stove and the initial process of your mouth salivating because you are hungry—just the visual or maybe the smell makes your mouth water in anticipation. This is the onset of your body's ability to produce digestive enzymes naturally. If you order takeout all the time, you aren't fully experiencing that vital step. Therefore, cooking at home has so many underestimated benefits. Also, when we eat in a rush or under stress, the process is compromised. Simplify things for your body and go back to rest and digest.

Our pancreas is also responsible for secreting digestive enzymes, but its output can be impacted by processed food or drink that promotes intestinal inflammation. That—along with potential other factors such as age, celiac disease, stress, medications, Crohn's, IBS, or diabetes—can lead to issues with digesting properly, and you may need more time to build up enzymes organically.

Overeating can also give your body more than it can handle. If you are lacking digestive enzymes for any reason, too much food at once will prevent your body from digesting it effectively. This is a classic food intolerance with uncomfortable symptoms like cramping and gas, which leads to nutritional deficiencies and the onset of GI disorders. Smaller meals may help improve the imbalance.

If you suspect that age, long-term medications, or stress, for example, have contributed to a lack of essential enzymes, talk to your doctor or a GI specialist about your symptoms, potential causes, and whether a supportive enzyme protocol might be a favorable course of action for you. However, it is possible for the body to replenish these enzymes with supportive dietary modifications, and I believe the best digestive enzymes are the ones our bodies make naturally. We improve, replace, and reinforce natural bodily functions by supporting the processes and eating more intact plant-based foods. Here are a couple of other things you can consider:

• Chew food longer—it benefits enzymatic activity.
• Do not drink liquid during meals, as it dilutes these enzymes.
• As always, keep away from processed foods, as these inflammatory foods will only create more of a burden in the form of a more acidic environment.
• Add in more foods that contain natural digestive enzymes, such as pineapples, mangos, papayas, honey, bananas, avocados, kefir, sauerkraut, kimchi, miso, kiwifruit, and ginger.
• Try apple cider vinegar (ACV), which is considered alkaline and helps with proper digestion. A little goes a long way, so please do not drink straight from the bottle. Mix no more than a tablespoon with eight ounces of water and sip slowly before a meal. This simple ritual will aid in digesting your food with natural enzymes and acetate.[91] Anecdotal evidence suggests many benefits associated with adding ACV to water, salads, and even the brining of pickles. Please note that this is not a miracle cure, and for some, ACV could exacerbate symptoms of an ulcer or GERD; it's also not suggested for anyone with low potassium levels.

UNDERSTANDING SUPPLEMENTS

Having annual checkups with and blood work done by a trusted doctor is essential for proactive care. I would consider supplementation only when advised because of a health necessity and imbalance.

Circumstances change, and we must adapt to our bodies and their needs. The most important take-home message regarding supplements is this: pay no attention to what supplements your friends, relatives, or gym buddies are taking for one thing or another. Many of these supplements are not regulated and are cheaply made. Your body and its needs are unique, so proper testing will help pinpoint deficiencies and any needed supplementation.

For example, taking hair growth supplements got me into trouble years back as excessive biotin (marked clearly on the bottle as 10,000 times the recommended daily allowance!) messed with my crucial bone turnover markers. When resorption happens at a higher rate than turnover, it leads to a decrease in bone mass. After stopping this extremely pricey and well-known supplement, my numbers were standard within three months. Further investigation uncovered limited evidence that biotin even benefits hair and nail growth.[92] I decided to stick to bananas, cauliflower, sweet potatoes, avocados, nuts, seeds, and legumes, as they are rich plant-based sources of biotin.

If you decide on nutritional supplementation, the following are tips for maximum efficient absorption:

- Do not take calcium with iron as they compete for absorption. Wait at least an hour in between them.
- Iron taken with vitamin C will increase iron absorption.
- Do not take B vitamins at night as they may keep you from getting a good night's sleep.
- Calcium and vitamin D need each other. Vitamin D is the carrier and boosts calcium absorption.
- If you have caffeine, wait an hour after consumption to take your vitamins. The tannins and caffeine will interfere with absorption, especially iron.
- If you have been diagnosed with celiac or suspect a gluten sensitivity, chances are you may have B12 deficiencies. B12 deficiencies go hand in hand with anemia and low iron levels.
- Water soluble vitamins (Bs, C, niacin, riboflavin, and biotin) dissolve in water and in our bodies, but the body cannot store them. Any excess will simply pass out of the body through the kidneys.
- A healthy gut is necessary for proper absorption of vital fat soluble vitamins (A, D, E, and K). They are not the easiest to digest and dietary fat is needed to dissolve, absorb, and store them for when the body needs access. On the other hand, since they are fat soluble, it is easier to absorb more than you really need. Anything in excess isn't removed by the kidneys once the need is met.

MAINTAIN YOUR BEAUTIFUL SKIN

Clean and clear skin goes beyond washing up with a mild cleanser and a dose of daily sunscreen. Caring for your skin and maintaining a youthful appearance requires the proper nutrients, hydration (so much hydration!), less stress, and plenty of sleep. Better food choices, like healthy fats containing compounds rich in zinc and vitamin E, protect our skin from harmful UV damage. Other nutrients like vitamin C aid in creating collagen, the main structural protein keeping our skin strong, healthy, and resilient. Plant-based foods containing beta-carotene convert into vitamin A in our body for that radiant glow. Amp up on beneficial omega-3s, which improve the skin barrier, sealing in moisture and keeping out irritants and toxins.

> **Load up on the good stuff! Here are great plant-based sources of all the nutrients discussed here.**
>
> - **Beta-carotene:** yellow, orange, and green leafy fruits and vegetables such as broccoli rabe, cantaloupe, sweet potatoes, and winter squash
> - **Omega-3s:** chia, flax, sunflower seeds, and walnuts
> - **Vitamin C:** bell peppers, broccoli, brussels sprouts, kiwi, oranges, pineapple, and spinach
> - **Vitamin E:** almonds, collard greens, peanuts, pumpkin, red bell peppers, and sunflower seeds
> - **Zinc:** legumes, nuts, oats, seeds, and tofu

The perks of plant nutrients and ample antioxidants are that they protect and hydrate on a cellular level and prevent free radicals from causing sun damage, premature wrinkles, eczema, acne, itchiness, and rashes. One of the many benefits you may have noticed during Reset is younger-looking, blemish-free skin. Would you like it to stay that way? If so, be careful about reintroducing certain skin-irritating foods. Everything in moderation, of course, but try to limit the following:

Alcohol: Excessive consumption of this toxin can wreak havoc on your delicate skin.

Blended coffee drinks: That Starbucks pit stop may seem like just the thing, but these kinds of drinks have way too much sugar. When we expose our bodies to excessive sugars, the inflammation associated will produce free radicals. Free radicals open the door to all sorts of health issues. When we consume plant-based foods, we support our immune system with many proactive antioxidants. Think of these antioxidants knocking those invaders right out of our bodies.

Butter and margarine (and by-products): These have too much saturated fat and the fillers and additives increase wrinkles.

Packaged snacks: Avoid crackers, chips, and cookies that use ingredients like butter, inflammatory oils, and cheese and cheese by-products. Excess amounts of fat, sugar, and salt will also create inflammation, cause water retention, and leave skin looking swollen.

Fried foods: Too many trans fats leave your skin vulnerable to harmful UV rays by breaking down collagen. In addition, clogged pores and acne are often exacerbated by these harmful oils. Ultraviolet A (UVA) radiation makes up 95 percent of UV rays and is responsible for aging our skin. All the more reason to wear that sunscreen. Ultraviolet B is the other 5 percent and is responsible for skin burning.

Packaged soups, sauces, and dressings: Making your own is so much better, and it's a snap too! In addition to the Reset condiments, sauces, and dips, Maintenance recipes worth keeping in your new rotation include Sweet Onion and White Bean Dip, Chili-Carrot Spread, and Verde Pico de Gallo. Furthermore, the Roasted Vegetables and Mushroom Stew and Black Lentil Minestrone are perfect comfort meals and must-tries!

Red meat: Beef contains the highest amount of advanced glycation end products (see AGEs).

In addition to paying attention to food choices, supportive self-care for vibrant looking skin that will stand the test of time requires soothing and calming routines. Taking time for yourself to gently wash your face without harsh chemicals is first on the list. Sleep, fresh air, clean sheets, moisturizer, sunscreen, and plenty of water are also standard rituals that will undoubtedly pay off. Relax, refresh, and renew with facials, a mani-pedi, and body massages to keep all that skin supple. What to do with all those papaya skins? Papaya is rich in papain, an enzyme that increases cell turnover. Just rub the flesh side of a peel over age spots on the face, hands, and chest and let it absorb for a quick at-home facial.

The Best Antiaging Plant-Based Foods

Avocados	Eggplants	Pomegranates
Bananas	Ground Flaxseeds	Spinach
Bell Peppers (red and yellow)	Kale	Sweet potatoes
	Lemons	Tomatoes
Blueberries	Nuts	Watercress
Broccoli	Papayas	Watermelon
Brussels Sprouts		

HISTAMINE AND POLYPHENOLS

So while you are putting in such great efforts to remove inflammatory foods, I encourage you to return to the idea that one size *does not* fit all. Through the practices of eliminating triggers and gaining awareness of how our bodies react to food, situations, and so on, we become better positioned to pinpoint where attention is needed.

Let's explore histamine and its role in our bodies. For example, we are often told to increase fermented foods in our diets if we suspect gut issues. Fermented foods have high levels of histamine that occur naturally. For some, that broad stroke of a brush for "best gut health" will not quickly solve problems across the board.

Histamine is a chemical compound stored in mast and other immune cells and is most known for its role during an allergic reaction. To protect the body, histamine works with the nerves to produce itching or hives. With food allergies, vomiting or diarrhea occurs. Even more severe is the likeliness of life-threatening anaphylaxis. Other functions of histamine are to trigger the regulation of stomach acid and to communicate messages to the brain for optimal cognitive functions. When the central nervous system is overloaded or compromised, this impairment can result in an overproduction of histamine, causing negative effects on cognitive, immune, and behavioral functions.

Histamine intolerance occurs when there is an overproduction of histamine or our body is unable to efficiently break it down due to a lack of the enzyme diamine oxidase (DAO). This enzyme is responsible for breaking down the histamine we take in from food. A lack of the enzyme is associated with meds, leaky gut, bacterial overgrowth, and an excess of histamine-rich foods. This imbalance affects normal body functions and expected responses, and symptoms include

- Cramping
- Digestive issues
- Dizziness
- Flushing
- Headaches
- High blood pressure
- Hives, rashes, itchy skin, and eczema
- Sudden excessive sweating

One of the most common causes of histamine intolerance is an imbalanced microbiome. This intolerance may lead to more severe ailments such as sleep disorders, low blood pressure, irregular heartbeat, and asthma.

Foods containing histamine are aged and fermented foods, alcohol (especially red wine), canned fish, dried fruit, eggplant, processed and smoked meats, shellfish, spinach, and tomatoes. These foods will feed the imbalance and make symptoms like congestion, headaches, fatigue, hives, or itching more uncomfortable.[93] Foods that can trigger histamine release are alcohol, bananas, beans, some citrus (lemons, limes, and oranges), food dyes, papaya, tomatoes, and nuts (walnuts, cashews, and peanuts), along with preservatives and additives.

To block or counteract the effects of too much histamine, we typically take histamine blockers called antihistamines (Benadryl, Claritin, and Zyrtec). It is common to take these medicines to quickly relieve allergy symptoms like hives, insect bites, and hay fever. If you deal with uncomfortable seasonal allergy responses, consider those trigger foods and avoid them when you know histamine levels are high—as this action will aid in alleviating short-term bothersome issues.

In addition, consider supportive dietary plant polyphenols. These naturally occurring compounds with antioxidant properties and natural antihistamine stabilizers counteract high levels of histamine. These stabilizing compounds are present in vitamin C–rich foods such as berries, broccoli, cauliflower, citrus fruits, and tropical fruits. Other sources are some beverages (coffee and tea), chocolate, flaxseeds, legumes, nuts, oils, olives, and spices. Yes, lemon can potentially trigger a histamine release or tame a reaction because it is also rich in polyphenolic compounds. One size does not fit all. You are your best judge in these situations.

These various polyphenolic compounds are also associated with reducing inflammation markers, improving insulin resistance, repairing cells, and protecting against oxidative stress to vital cells. More reasons to eat plant-based foods. Polyphenols should be the most abundant antioxidant source in our diet. These micronutrients are easily attainable with more plant-based foods but are also available through superfood supplementation. Watch the sourced manufacturer though, as many of these supplements (nonorganic superfood powders) are full of fillers, artificial sweeteners, and potential pesticides that bring about more stress to the digestive tract.

THE THYMUS GLAND

This gland, just in front of and above your heart, is a significant player in supporting the immune system. The thymus fights infection by producing T cells, which are crucial for maintaining optimal immunity. Once T cells are established, they travel to your lymph nodes, where they act against inflammation and disease. The gland functions at its peak when we are young and weakens as we age. We cannot reverse the aging process, but we can support immune functions with these actions and nutrients:

- Avoiding sugar at all costs (sugar depresses immune responses)
- Plant-based micronutrients (herbs, garlic, ginger, and turmeric)
- Quality sleep

- Selenium (Brazil nuts, broccoli, greens, peas, and potatoes)
- Vitamin A (mango; papaya; apricots; and yellow, red, and green leafy veggies)
- Vitamin C (kiwi, citrus, strawberries, brussels sprouts, and potatoes)
- Zinc (pumpkin seeds, legumes, and seeds)

> Another way to support the health of the thymus is to activate it. Using your four fingertips or the side of your fist, tap up and down two to three inches along the base of the sternum (around the third rib) to effectively stimulate the gland. Take slow breaths and tap for fifteen to twenty seconds.

If we manage and support cell functions throughout the body, it is possible to dispose of old, damaged cells and replace them with a renewed restorative version. I'm game! This new environment and foundation you've created are now better equipped to provide you with the most favorable outcome. Tap into that renewal process and keep all immune responses supported and synchronized in your favor.

THE THYROID GLAND

The thyroid gland (not to be confused with the thymus gland) is located at the front of the neck. Its function is to convert oxygen and calories to energy. Our cells depend on the thyroid to hormonally regulate our metabolism. Most autoimmune thyroid illnesses usually present with underlying inflammation triggers such as chronic stress, gluten sensitivity, an imbalanced ratio of good to bad gut bacteria, Epstein-Barr virus, or high levels of environmental toxin exposure (such as glyphosate in the weed killer Roundup).

Optimizing thyroid hormones can tremendously benefit and address food sensitivities and play a significant role in maintaining the intestinal lining. Less stress, exercise, and clean food ensure essential functions. Plant-based food sources to strengthen the thyroid are avocados, selenium and tyrosine from Brazil nuts, mushrooms, pumpkin seeds, and walnuts. Zinc from lentils, nuts, and seeds are also supportive foods. Iodine is a fundamental component of the thyroid hormone, and sources like dulse, kelp, nori, and healthy amounts of iodized salt will protect this precious balance.

If you are struggling with hypothyroidism issues, be mindful that large amounts of foods like soy and raw cruciferous vegetables can block the absorption of iodine in the thyroid. If you are diagnosed with hyperthyroidism or hypothyroidism, and taking prescribed medication, consuming excess kelp, iodine, and selenium may hinder the proper absorption of drugs or deliver them in excess, which is not beneficial. Be aware that gluten sensitivity is a major trigger for those struggling with Hashimoto's. Avoiding gluten can help keep this disease well managed while balancing these hormones.[94]

ISSUES THAT MAY NEED EXTRA SUPPORT

Adrenal Fatigue Syndrome

Imagine overloading all the circuits in your home with too much electricity, more than your circuit board can handle. What happens next? Darkness. We've all been in situations when—overworked or overstimulated—our own lights go out, and we are left scratching our heads, wondering why.

As discussed in part 1, the HPA axis regulates responses to stress. When it is overworked from stress and inflammation, we experience chaos. In the adrenal glands (the *A* part of HPA), which produce cortisol in response to stress, this can culminate in adrenal fatigue. Symptoms of adrenal fatigue include sleep issues, weight problems, compromised detoxification, tiredness, infertility, PMS, heart palpitations, food sensitivities, low libido, and brain fog.

Just like the circuitry in your house, the adrenal glands need maintenance to function properly. What happens if you leave plump, juicy grapes out in the hot sun? You'll end up with dry, shriveled raisins. Depleting the adrenal glands has the same consequences. Dried out, overworked, and exhausted is no way to go through life when renewal is available. Revisit the important functions of hormones and the HPA axis in the Repair section. Equally supportive is being consistent in your responsibility to the self-care acts mentioned in the Be Aware section, as prioritizing rituals for more peaceful moments is part of your resilient foundation. Your commitment to balance and better habits will support this rejuvenation.

AGEs

Advanced glycation end products (AGEs) are harmful compounds formed when protein or fat combine with sugar in the bloodstream. This process is called glycation. Animal-derived foods that are high in fat and protein, such as meats (especially red meats), are prone to AGE formation through cooking. AGEs are present even more with charred, overcooked meats. They are found in fried eggs, butter, cream cheese, margarine, mayonnaise, oils, and nuts. Other common sources are sugary foods and highly processed and prepackaged products.

If you do not consume high amounts of AGEs, your body will eliminate them naturally. If you do a good amount of grilling, frying, or toasting at high temperatures, these harmful compounds will accumulate in your body. As you learn more about the importance of plant-based food choices, remember that certain convenience foods may be aging you more than you know.

Bone Health

Osteoporosis is an autoimmune disease that causes bones to become weak and brittle. It is often undiagnosed until there is significant damage to the bones and is often associated with those diagnosed with celiac and gluten sensitivities or type 1 and type 2 diabetes. Digestive and GI disorders lead to malabsorption issues and, thus, insufficient nutrients for proper bone growth. An overly acidic environment and too much inflammation also contribute to bone loss. The body wants to heal and correct the overly acidic habitat, so it tries to neutralize with minerals, specifically calcium, which is pulled from the bones. Low calcium, hormonal imbalances, thyroid issues, diet, eating disorders, and age are among the top common causes of bone loss.

Calcium Considerations

Healthy bones thrive on calcium in conjunction with other minerals to form hard crystals. This gives our bones much-needed strength and structure to carry us through life—literally! Ninety-nine percent of the body's calcium is found in our skeletal structure, so it's important that we consume and absorb this mineral effectively. We are often told that calcium must come from dairy, yet dairy can cause acidic reactions, which of course we want to avoid. If your body is okay with dairy occasionally, a slice of hard parmesan cheese can offer a hefty dose of calcium while being easily digestible due to its low amount of lactase. If you choose not to consume dairy or if you believe dairy may be causing you discomfort, you may need to adjust your calcium intake accordingly.

The good news is that you can increase calcium intake with plant-based options. Try sautéing, boiling, or steaming vegetables like broccoli, turnip greens, dandelion greens, mustard greens, and kale, which can be absorbed most efficiently by these cooking methods (see Steamed Vegetables). Baked Seaweed Snacks are also a supportive way to improve calcium absorption. Tahini and beans will boost your calcium intake (see Collard Green Wraps). Chia seeds, edamame, fortified plant-based milk, tempeh, and tofu are also excellent sources. Figs and rhubarb contain calcium and other bone-building nutrients and minerals like phosphorus, potassium, vitamin K, and iron. Blackstrap molasses is the heavy hitter here. Just two tablespoons offer 400 milligrams of calcium. I like to substitute molasses for honey in baked recipes (see Anytime Bars). You get the sweetness and a warm, robust flavor in addition to this much-needed mineral.

Reduced HCL production affects the amount of protein and calcium we can absorb and can interfere with bone metabolism. Incomplete protein metabolism can cause deficiencies and imbalanced intestinal gut flora. Also be mindful of sugar intake, as increased consumption results in the urinary excretion of calcium, magnesium, and potassium, all essential bone nutrients. In addition, opt for low sodium convenience foods, as too much sodium interferes with calcium absorption. On the other hand, vitamins D and C boost absorption. Sit in the sun to absorb your daily dose of vitamin D and eat a delicious salad containing an array of bone-building nutrients (see Thai Chopped Salad).

As the causes of osteoporosis are varied, keep in mind that there is no one-size-fits-all course of action, but supportive measures are available: a clean diet, exercise in the form of weight-bearing activities, and minimizing stress to help optimize hormonal functions.

Medication is vital for some with this diagnosis, but timing is also a major consideration for starting any drugs. I am personally familiar with having to start bisphosphonates, but I only did so when I fully understood the commitment and possible side effects. Long-term use caused me distress, so I sought professionals who respected my fears. I also waited two years and got my gut, immune, and hormone responses in better balance to support the therapy with extremely positive results.

Celiac Disease

Celiac disease is a chronic immune disorder that is triggered by consuming gluten. As mentioned, gluten sensitivity is one of the most prevalent and common inflammatory disorders that can cause long-lasting digestive issues. Common symptoms include pain in the abdomen, achy joints, diarrhea, heartburn, indigestion, headaches, fatigue, and nausea. Long-term complications are skin rashes, bone loss, malnutrition, slow-growth, and delayed puberty. Related conditions are hypothyroidism, malabsorption, anemia, leaky gut, and peripheral neuropathy. Some people have little to no symptoms (silent celiac) but may complain of anxiety, acid reflux, or bloating. These issues may not seem worrisome, but they can still do damage to the small intestine.[95]

Diagnosing celiac disease can be tricky. You can take a blood test, but it requires that you be on a gluten-containing regime for close-to-accurate testing. Consequently, false-positive results are common. Conclusive testing could come from a genetic marker test for human leukocyte antigen genes. A gastrointestinal specialist might also test intestinal villi with a biopsy, as these hairlike projections that aid digestion in the small intestine can be damaged and potentially atrophied by celiac disease.

Gluten hides in many everyday convenience items in addition to less obvious sources, like tea bags (sealed with wheat starch), energy bars, ice cream, and frozen desserts. Gluten can also be found in beverages, daily supplements, hygiene products, medications, and the glue on envelopes. Certified gluten-free products are more regulated and held to a higher standard, so look for foods that can claim this.

Read labels and listen to your body. If you have a first-degree family member with celiac, your chances increase, and you should consider DNA testing for a conclusive result. If you suspect anything, trust your gut and seek help.

The Menopause Journey

Perimenopause, menopause, and postmenopause: what they mean and what you can do to alleviate any symptoms is vital information to most women over the age of forty. Or—should we be more mindful at an earlier age?

It is often seen as a curse, and why not? When women experience a decline in estrogen, symptoms such as mood swings, night sweats, vaginal atrophy, headaches, irregular periods, and the end of periods and the reproductive years hit hard. They are faced with a new unchartered phase of their lives. No one seems to want to be around them unless, of course, they joke and make fun of themselves for sweating in forty-five-degree weather. This trip is different for all women, so hold on tight.

As you know, hormones are the body's chemical messengers, and the ones we're interested in here are the sex hormones: estrogen and progesterone (and to a lesser extent, testosterone). The endocrine system regulates these hormones (and others), controlling mood, hunger, growth, sugar levels, reproduction, and puberty. But hormonal balance is affected by internal and external disruptors. The right foods play an essential role in regulating hormones, but external endocrine disruptors that mimic estrogen range from plastics, canned foods, shampoos, creams, makeup, and air fresheners to name a few.

In a nutshell, and in a perfect world, the natural menopausal transition would be as follows. Estrogen levels start to decline with age. Irregular periods and less responsive egg development note the beginning of perimenopause. Shifting into menopause means estrogen and progesterone levels continue to decline and ovaries stop releasing an egg once a month. A person is considered postmenopausal immediately after periods have ceased for more than a year.

Though this process sounds simple enough, many women have a difficult time with menopause due to fluctuating hormones. Polycystic ovary syndrome, painful periods, endometriosis, and infertility are on the rise in younger women. Could these "common symptoms" be a precursor to a not-so-healthy transition to menopause? Could endocrine disruptors throw us into early-onset perimenopause and open the door to premature osteoporosis, depression, autoimmune disease, heart disease, and cancers?

Removing inflammatory foods and adding fresh, organic produce is a game changer and the first step in preventive care. Hydration is always important at any age. The next level includes external factors. Start by eliminating toxic chemicals from your everyday environment: avoid additives and preservatives; buy chemical-free cosmetics, cleaning products, and bug sprays; and store your food in glass instead of plastic containers. Toxins can also be people in your life, a job situation, finances, too much worrying, and a constant survival mode that creates chronic anxiety. This fight-or-flight mode affects the function of the thyroid and the immune response, metabolism, and reproductive system.

Perhaps you're already there and wondering how to alleviate the symptoms you're experiencing. If they are severe, consult a medical professional, preferably one who specializes in menopause. In addition to homing in on internal and external factors, a little TLC goes a long way at times. Focus on what makes you feel *your* best, not anyone else's. Consider gentle self-care practices, such as a nature walk, infrared sauna session, facial, massage, or just a good night's sleep. You cannot stop the aging process, but you can find your balance. Embrace the beauty within and shine on the outside because you are beautiful and strong.

Sustainable lifestyle modifications and practices that leave you feeling centered most days is the goal. Focus on happy moments and breathe. Perfection is not attainable, so be more accepting of the wonderful person you already are. Get informed and appreciate the journey. When you get there, you get there.

Migraines

If you experience chronic migraines, you probably already know that the cause can be difficult to pinpoint. This debilitating pain commonly occurs in one hemisphere of the head and can last hours to multiple days. Medications can help, but generally these are taken at the onset of pain and are not preventive. In addition, any medication will not address the root cause of the issue. An elimination diet is a great place to start, so with Reset 90/10, you're already on your way! As you begin adding back in eliminated foods, keep a journal to note what provokes migraines.

Uncovering triggers is rewarding, as I've witnessed many clients living with the debilitating pain and isolation a migraine delivers. Culprits I found with one client were gum with probable preservatives like butylated hydroxytoluene (BHT) and the pressure gum chewing puts on the joint of the lower jaw. Highly processed soy products were an eye-opener for another client, as she often relied on protein bars and quick meals. Examples are plant-based soy burgers and foods with isolated soy protein or soy flours, which may contain soy isoflavones (an organic compound considered an endocrine disruptor when consumed in large amounts). When buying soy sauce, look for brands that are "naturally brewed," which means they are made from a special fermentation process—otherwise, they are chemically processed. It is also important for those with sensitivities to know that soy sauce contains wheat.

Other likely triggers include specific types of artificial sweeteners, preservatives, and additives in everyday products. Food triggers might be additives, aged cheeses, artificial sweeteners, eggs, dairy, MSG, nitrates, nuts, onions, orange juice, processed or smoked foods, tomatoes, wheat, and yeast. Watch for synonymous names of MSG, including "monosodium salt," "monosodium glutamate," "sodium glutamate," and "monohydrate."

Magnesium deficiency is commonly reported in those who suffer from migraines. Exceptional sources of magnesium include avocados, bananas, brown rice, dark chocolate, dark leafy greens, legumes, lima beans, nuts, pumpkin seeds, and tuna.

Getting energy from the right foods is a positive step, but emotional factors can also have an influence on migraines. Stress activates an influx of hormones, primarily cortisol from the adrenal glands. More and more cortisol pumping from our adrenal glands is the beginning stage of adrenal fatigue and is often associated with migraines (see Adrenal Fatigue Syndrome). Other common causes could be skipping meals, poor sleep habits, caffeine, alcohol, bright lights, and loud noises.

Hormones, as we have learned, are the body's chemical messengers. Estrogen normally fluctuates during the menstrual cycle, but the trigger of a premenstrual migraine typically occurs when estrogen and progesterone are lowest. Supportive therapies for migraine relief that you might consider are acupuncture, nerve stimulation, stress management, yoga, essential oils, and relaxation training.

Oxidative Stress and Insulin Resistance

Oxidative stress in the body results from a biological inability to repair and detoxify. Insulin controls the amount of glucose in your blood, and when cells don't respond well to insulin, they can't use the energy properly. This leads to the pancreas producing more insulin and results in excess glucose being stored, which increases abdominal fat in a vicious cycle. This is where too much of a good thing comes into play. The constant release of stress hormones like cortisol and adrenaline makes it harder for insulin to perform properly. An overabundance of free radicals and a lack of superior antioxidant activity leads to damaged cells and proteins and DNA breakdown—what is called oxidative stress. This insulin resistance and the bodies failure to detoxify plays a pivotal role in the development of diabetes, obesity, cardiovascular health, and a healthful metabolism. Examining the correlation between oxidative stress and insulin resistance can lead to improvements of long-term health.

An appropriate diet rich in antioxidants will likely decrease oxidation and unwanted spikes in blood sugar. Consider also eating smaller meals throughout the day to keep insulin levels balanced. Intact forms of fruits and vegetables aid in the detoxification process of removing excess hormones from the body. Over time, excess toxins compromise our liver, adrenal glands, thyroid, kidneys, and other vital organs. The efficient release of insulin from the pancreas results in less visceral fat, better cell function, and less inflammation.[96]

The whole body is connected, and this is clear when looking at a couple of other potential problems associated with insulin. The thyroid controls metabolism, which is the chemical reactions within the body's cells that break down food into energy. If this doesn't function properly, there is likely a blood sugar imbalance and possibly insulin resistance.[97]

In addition, food sensitivities and the connection to insulin-resistant polycystic ovary syndrome (PCOS) are worth mentioning. Lifestyle choices that create chronic stress could negatively influence food choices, sleep patterns, and adrenal balance. Could all the above turn our hormones upside down and be a feasible link to insulin resistance?[98]

Here are the best ways to support stable insulin production and usage:

Get proper sleep. Wind down and repair. Turn lights down low in the evening to help set your circadian rhythm. Our circadian rhythm is the natural cycle of behavioral, physical, and mental changes that follow a twenty-four-hour internal clock in our brains. Our physiology and behaviors are regulated by cycles of alertness and sleepiness that respond to changes in our environment. No computer, phone, or television one to two hours before bed, as these bright screens impair a good night's sleep, which in addition to causing you to be tired the next day, also contributes to weight gain.

Stress less. What's eating you? Let it go. Various emotional and mental stressors affect the amount of cortisol released into the body and specific organs.

Clean up your diet. Focus on organic, fiber-rich, and unprocessed foods. Watch out for gluten-free products loaded with starches that mimic gluten if you are gluten-free or have sensitivities, as they tend to spike blood sugar. Also, avoid refined carbs and products with corn, soy, and refined sugars. Buy organic whenever possible to avoid crops sprayed with pesticides.

Hydrate. Our bodies need water to survive. Water helps regulate body temperatures, remove waste, deliver nutrients to cells, and keep organs functioning correctly.

Eliminate toxins. Whenever possible, get rid of chemical cleaning products, air fresheners, perfume, and candles. Eliminate sources of mold, nitrates, pesticides, and mercury. These toxins can easily alter our endocrine system.

Exercise. The benefits of exercise are enormous. Grab a friend and take a walk to reduce stress. Yoga, Pilates, and other forms of low-impact exercise are easy on your body and support strength and flexibility as well as healthy cardiovascular function. Nothing excessive, as too much exercise may inflame adrenals, raise cortisol to a dangerous level, drive inflammatory responses, and lead to a decrease in energy. Believe it or not, excessive exercise could be what keeps many active people, especially women, from dropping those extra few pounds.

Decrease inflammation. Chronic inflammation leads to belly fat and is seen primarily in poor diets. As seen throughout this book, inflammation opens the door to many diseases.

SPIRIT

GET HELP FROM PRACTITIONERS

If uncomfortable or concerning symptoms linger and you have that gut feeling that more care is needed, follow your instincts and inquire with a professional. In my journey, I saw many doctors and heard many different opinions. This was frustrating at times, but for me, ultimately even the not-so-supportive visits turned into learning experiences. You may have to put some time into research and trial and error, but the right professional will come along.

Look for a specialist who is truly supportive, encouraging, and empathic to your unique situation. This could be a gynecologist who

Alternatives to Long-Term Medications

Taking prescribed medication for longer than three months is considered long term.

For example, treating chronic lower back pain with painkillers is a ritual not uncommon in our world. But taking these meds can lead to difficulties beyond the physical nature of the pain. Dependence on painkillers may cause depression, addiction, anxiety, and difficulty sleeping, and while that may not sound so bad, those symptoms can have long-reaching effects.[101]

We need a new perspective when it comes to long-term medications. As Saray Stancic, an infectious disease doctor, noted:

> What if all physicians everywhere joined together and spoke up for the clear and universal power of lifestyle medicine? This would be a miracle. It could be the catalyst for a sweeping shift in how we define true health care and could add what is missing so that our system can focus on preserving health, not only treating sickness. In order to turn the tide of chronic disease and the epidemic of illnesses such as obesity, autoimmune disorders, diabetes, and the stress that goes along with them, we must evolve. Doctors and patients alike need to embrace a paradigm shift. Right now we're passive and powerless—convinced that our genes define us, food choices don't really matter, and prescription drugs will save us. Truly, we can only take control of our personal health outcomes by optimizing all aspects of lifestyle.

Are there alternatives to long-term meds? What are the implications of these drugs? Is there a different avenue?

Can you make changes with diet, exercise, stress reduction, therapy, and supplementation? Can you get a second or third opinion? Ask questions and gather information so you can make informed decisions about what's best for you.

Though alternative modalities might not work for everyone, they should be a place to start, as they can more effectively uncover the root cause of the issue.[102] Therapies like yoga, nutritional support, or lifestyle modifications could be offered as an alternate route. Reducing inflammatory responses through elimination of refined sugars and carbs. What if the pain was related to your chair at work or your shoes, excess exercise, or stress?

specializes in menopause, an endocrinologist, a GI specialist, an integrative health coach, or your trusted general practitioner. Whole-body wellness sometimes takes a team of professionals thinking outside the box and advocating a broader scope of treatments. If that's the case for you, know that you are worth it!

Remember, you should always feel comfortable with what is decided on your behalf. You are your own best advocate when you stay on top of your health with the proper balance, awareness, and education. Pull that knowledge out of your back pocket whenever in doubt and keep your "circle of life" plate balanced. Every aspect of your life is going to support excellent health.

GRASPING SELF-CARE

One of the most challenging aspects I find with many clients is structuring time for oneself. Engaging in self-care is a struggle even I face with guilt on occasion. At times, me-time is nowhere on my agenda, but that hurdle, like every other hurdle, is one I work to remove so I can stay happy, healthy, and resilient.

Downtime can mean many different engaging activities. Something as simple as a nap or sleeping in on the weekend can do wonders for relaxing and refreshing the spirit. Never underestimate the benefits of a nice long soak in the tub. On the other hand, signing up for energizing swing dance lessons alone or with a partner could work wonders on your morale, confidence, and mood.

Self-care might include revisiting the thought of transforming your bedroom into the sleep oasis you've always dreamed of, creating a place you look forward to properly resting in. In addition, a project like this could also help with decluttering.

My dog, Dug, is a beautiful example of love that holds no boundaries. Pets give unconditional love and are known to reduce stress, decrease blood pressure, offer companionship, and increase opportunities to be outside with nature, exercise, and socialize. That mutt helps me check off many self-care boxes!

Revisit strategies that bring you joy and implement these routines regularly. Take a time-out, get yourself back to an appropriate energy level, and continue evolving with joy, purpose, and peace of mind.

HITTING A PLATEAU WITH WEIGHT LOSS

When clients are in the Maintenance stage, feeling better about their choices and noticing less inflammation in their bodies, I often get asked about healthy weight loss as this journey continues.

Hitting a weight loss plateau is perfectly normal, and it's no reason to get discouraged in this journey. Yes, you have been putting your best effort in, but plateaus are normal and essential to weight loss. Do not let these frustrations cause reckless behavior in the quest for optimal health. Understanding that other factors such as behavioral, hormonal, or environmental conditions may also influence weight loss will enlighten you and shift the thought process into a more positive light.

Behavioral: Are you becoming too consumed with an unrealistic number? Are you enjoying your food and the changes you are experiencing? Be wary of becoming too restrictive with your food and exercise choices. Even something as simple as expecting change too soon can discourage the most focused individuals.

Hormonal: It is normal for the metabolism to slow down after weight loss, but it is also possible to give your metabolism a boost.

Environmental: Are you under stress? Try breathing, massage, or other forms of stress management. Also, ensure you're getting the right amount of exercise (not too much or too little) and adequate sleep. How is your mental clarity—can you recognize, understand, and organize your thoughts clearly? For more focus and clear perception, give attention to self-care, goal planning, harmony, gratitude, and staying connected, not only with yourself but with loved ones and genuine people. As you bring in the positive, remove the excess that burdens your thoughts and physical space. Hold on to what matters and imagine your life with less confusion and doubt. Conscious consideration to simplicity comes with amazing benefits.

Let's address why a plateau happens. A plateau eventually occurs on every weight loss journey. You may be eating mindfully and exercising regularly, but your efforts have become stagnant. Now is the time to change the approach by either cutting calories (within reason); looking at habits, portions, and processed foods (are they sneaking back in?); or reassessing physical activity. Also, always check in with emotional responses and stressors that may cause you to hold it all in or comfort yourself with food. Instead, let it go, take a walk, call a friend, and find a distraction that makes you happy.

If you are confident with your goals and want to reassess your current situation with more attention to charging up your metabolism, let's make adjustments!

- More activity: weight training, meditation, and Pilates
- Metabolism (thyroid) boosters: Plant-based protein such as beans, legumes, and nuts
- Mineral-rich foods (iron, calcium, selenium): seaweed, avocado, nuts and seeds, cruciferous vegetables, spirulina, and berries
- Spicy foods: if they don't give you discomfort

HOLDING ON TO HAPPINESS

I am and will always be a work in progress. I believe I am a nurturer at heart, but these days I have proudly moved caring for myself to the top of my list. Digging deep and looking at external stressors made me realize that giving my body a break was my best course of action. That involved eliminating foods that were not digesting correctly, excessive exercise, sugar, and chronic stress. Pinpointing my triggers and eliminating inflammation helped me have less overall anxiety, and I no longer feel the need to be "on" twenty-four hours a day.

I have made significant strides in my health with more awareness about how I feel and finding the time to care for myself. Self-care requires not only food, water, and exercise. A well-rounded human being needs quality time to align their overall spirit, eliminate stress, find joy, and hold on to happiness.

This journey is different for all of us, but we all want to feel good and be able to live our best lives. Food is essential, and with this guide I hope you will be able to follow a nutritious and sustainable path to health. The right food—along with healthy relationships, proper exercise, acts of self-care, a fulfilling career, and a spiritual practice—sustains our body, mind, and soul and allows us to thrive.

Like every other ideology, the Reset program is based on observation and experience. The field of evidence-based scientific study can be confusing because one study proves something while another disproves it. The variables change daily, as do our environments and situations. Giving yourself hope and empowerment through self-care may not always have scientific studies to back it up, but let the evidence speak for itself. How do those activities make you feel? I have witnessed many clients make transformations they never thought possible. With this ripple effect, we can get closer to the root of pain and illness.

While we all strive to be our best, remember, as Voltaire reputedly said, "Perfect is the enemy of good." This journey is about finding a reasonable balance, as getting caught up in perfection will only hinder your progress. That which we manifest is before us, so keep all your good intentions going and hold on to whatever makes you happy.

PART FOUR

The Recipes

CHAPTER 13

Reset 90/10 Recipes

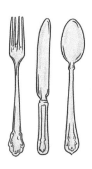

BREAKFAST

CELERY JUICE
MAKES 1 SERVING

I have been drinking 16 ounces of celery juice daily for close to seven years now, and while there are many theories on how to consume it or what to add, I find that straight celery juice first thing in the morning on an empty stomach is the way to go.

- 1 large bunch celery (see notes)

Clean the celery by cutting off the bottom base and the tips (if browned). Wash the separated stalks in clean water to remove any dirt and debris.

If using a juicer, feed the celery through your juicer and drink immediately.

If using a blender, cut up the celery and put it in a blender with about ¼ cup water. If you are unsure how powerful your blender is, cut the celery into smaller pieces. Blend on the highest speed for about 1 minute until the consistency is smooth. Place a clean nut milk bag or cheesecloth over a large bowl, strain the contents of the blender, and squeeze the celery juice through the bag using your hands.

NOTES: I see some sad-looking celery in the supermarkets. Look for healthy, light-green, thick stalks to get the most flavor and juice. The thickness and size will determine the amount of juice; you may have to use a little more for a 16-ounce glass.

If you'd rather not make juice every day, you can double or triple this recipe. Store what you don't drink right away in an airtight mason jar in the refrigerator. Just keep in mind that anything stored longer than 72 hours will lose a significant amount of nutrients and may develop unhealthy bacteria. Or you can freeze the extra and then thaw it in the refrigerator overnight as needed. You may notice changes in the color of frozen juices due to normal oxidation.

Other Fresh Juices

You can make juices with other fruits and vegetables in a juicer or blender, but you'll get various results. Cucumbers (see Hydrating Fruits and Vegetables in part 2) contain more water than a beet, for example. If experimenting, note that you may have to use some water when blending certain types of produce.

WARM LEMON WATER
MAKES 1 SERVING

This may be the simplest—and most effective—recipe ever.

- 1 teaspoon lemon juice
- 8 ounces warm water

Stir the lemon juice into the water. Drink immediately.

NOTES: Keep some not-from-concentrate bottled lemon juice on hand just in case you run out of lemons.

Also, if you get into using your juicer for more than just celery juice, try juicing a bag of lemons (cut off most of the peel first) and storing the juice in a mason jar in the refrigerator. It comes in handy for flavoring water, enhancing a bowl of soup, or adding a tasty zest to salad dressing.

ENERGY FRUIT SMOOTHIE
MAKES 1 SERVING

This is still my favorite part of the morning. An effective time-saving tip for smoothie making is as follows: if you are using a single-use blender cup, set up your smoothie the night before with everything except your frozen bananas. It's okay if your other frozen fruit thaws out overnight. Make the frozen banana the only thing you need to add to your blender cup in the morning.

- ½ cup juice of choice (freshly juiced fruits and vegetables, carrot juice, coconut water)
- ½ cup water or aloe vera juice (see notes)
- 2 tablespoons ground hempseed, ground flaxseed, or protein powder (see notes)
- ½ frozen or fresh banana (frozen will make it thicker)
- Handful of frozen fruit chunks (berries, mangos, pineapple, dark cherries)
- Half a handful of fresh cilantro
- Half a handful of raw baby spinach, baby kale, or sprouts (optional, see notes)
- 1 tablespoon barley grass powder or spirulina (optional)

Put all the ingredients in a high-speed blender and blend until well combined and smooth. Enjoy immediately.

NOTES: If using aloe vera juice, look for 100% pure juice, otherwise you will have a very bitter-tasting smoothie.

Please see recommended protein powder brands under Pantry Nice-to-Haves, as there are many gastrointestinal side effects associated with brands containing whey (dairy), sugar alcohols, additives, fillers, and preservatives.

Baby greens provide the most nutrient-dense outcome and are the easiest greens to digest during the Reset phase, so they are highly recommended for your morning smoothie. Use whatever you have on hand.

Utilize all those banana skins! You can make a liquid fertilizer for your plants by simply soaking banana peels for three to four days in a jar filled with water. I typically soak peels from four to five bananas in a two-quart jar, but you can modify the amount depending on the size of your jar. Bananas contain potassium, nitrogen, phosphorus, and magnesium—perfect for healthy plant growth.

APPLE PIE SMOOTHIE
MAKES 1 SERVING

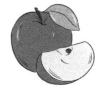

If you are hit by a sweet craving, this is a nice treat for an afternoon slump. Being more conscious of your cravings helps you satiate them mindfully.

- 1 frozen banana
- 1 apple, peeled and cored
- Dash of vanilla extract
- Sprinkle of apple pie spice
- ⅓ to ½ cup coconut, oat, or flax milk
- 2 tablespoons ground hempseed or ground flaxseed, or 1 serving protein powder (optional, but encouraged)
- Dash of maple syrup (optional)

Put all the ingredients in a high-speed blender and blend until well combined and smooth. Start with ⅓ cup milk for a thicker consistency, and if you want a thinner texture, add a bit more milk.

LUNCH AND DINNER

SPAGHETTI SQUASH WITH NONDAIRY CHEESE SAUCE
MAKES 2 TO 3 SERVINGS
CHEESE SAUCE MAKES ABOUT 2 CUPS

This is the ultimate comfort food for the health minded. The cheese sauce is something I encourage you to bookmark and use on many different foods, such as gluten-free or plant-based pasta, asparagus, Baked Potatoes, lasagna (after Reset), or brussels sprouts (after Reset)—the opportunities to enjoy it are endless!

- 1 medium spaghetti squash

NONDAIRY CHEESE SAUCE:

- 2 medium white or sweet potatoes, cooked, peeled, and diced
- 1 medium carrot, cooked, peeled, and diced
- 1 to 2 cloves Roasted Garlic (optional, use only if it doesn't upset your stomach)
- ½ teaspoon ground paprika
- Handful of fresh basil, or 1 teaspoon dried basil
- 1 teaspoon ground oregano
- ½ teaspoon ground turmeric
- 1 tablespoon lemon juice

- ½ teaspoon sea salt
- ¼ to ⅓ cup nutritional yeast, plus extra for serving
- ⅓ to ½ cup vegetable stock or nut milk

Preheat the oven to 400°F.

Cut off both ends of the squash. Cut the squash in half lengthwise and scoop out the seeds.

Line a baking pan with parchment paper. Sprinkle a little salt on the inside of the squash and turn it upside down, so the skin faces up. Add ¾ cup water to the pan and roast for 45 minutes or until fork tender. Remove from the oven, flip the squash carefully to release the steam, and let both halves sit for 10 to 15 minutes to cool off.

Use a fork to rake the squash lengthwise, making "spaghetti noodles." If the strands are not coming off easily, that usually means it needs to cook longer.

To make the cheese sauce, put all the sauce ingredients in a high-speed blender and blend on high for 30 seconds. Begin with ⅓ cup stock and add more as needed until it's the perfect thick and creamy texture. Also, begin with ¼ cup nutritional yeast and add more to taste. Do not overblend, as it will become too gooey. Season with salt and pepper to taste.

After roasting the squash and making the cheese sauce, combine them by folding the cheese sauce into the squash strands. Sprinkle with extra nutritional yeast, if you like, and serve.

NOTE: Consider doubling the cheese sauce recipe and freezing the extra to add to other meals.

SAVORY VEGETABLE CAKES
MAKES 6 TO 7 CAKES

These savory cakes can be the vehicle for a delicious salad or a great pairing with soup, curry, or stew. My favorite way to have them is with avocado, baby sprouts, sliced red onion, and diced pickled beets or radishes. Whipped Tahini Sauce would also complement these savory vegetables. It's a wonderful way to change up the rotation of your vegetables, as any root vegetables will work in this recipe. Be creative, have fun, and use up your veggies!

- 2 tablespoons olive, coconut, or avocado oil
- 2 tablespoons ground flaxseed
- ⅓ cup water
- 4 cups sweet potato, carrots, butternut squash, or a combination, grated (see notes)
- 1 small red onion or 2 shallots, chopped (see notes)
- ¼ cup buckwheat flour
- ½ teaspoon baking powder
- ¼ teaspoon salt
- ½ teaspoon ground spicy or smoked paprika
- ½ teaspoon ground sweet paprika
- ½ teaspoon ground coriander or cumin

Preheat the oven to 375°F. Line a baking sheet with parchment paper and lightly coat it with the oil (pump sprays work well too).

In a large bowl, create the flax egg by combining the flaxseed and water and letting it sit for 5 minutes. Fold in the grated vegetables and onion.

In a small bowl, mix the flour, baking powder, salt, spicy paprika, sweet paprika, and coriander. Add the dry ingredients to the grated vegetable mixture. Mix with your hands until well combined and sticking together.

Make 6 to 7 (5-inch) disks using ½ cup of the mixture for each cake, pushing in the edges while patting down the middle until you have a well-formed disk. Place all the cakes on the parchment paper and bake for 20 minutes. Flip and bake for an additional 15 minutes. The vegetable cakes should have a golden-brown and crispy exterior when done.

Season with salt and pepper to taste. Serve hot, and freeze any extras.

NOTES: After the Reset phase, you can add grated napa cabbage to the veggie mix.

During Reset, onions should be used only if they do not bother your stomach.

ROASTED VEGETABLES
MAKES 2 OR MORE SERVINGS (SEE NOTES)

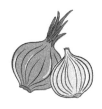

You're in for a treat when roasting vegetables. Chopping up and peeling what you have may require prep time, but the result is something everyone will enjoy (even the pickiest eaters). Remember that after Reset, veggies like broccoli, cauliflower, and brussels sprouts can be added back in.

During Reset, try potatoes (look for all different colors for a diversity of nutrients), butternut squash, green beans, asparagus, celery root, turnips, beets, summer squash, and even tomatoes. When serving roasted vegetables as a meal, a simple salad is always encouraged as a side. Use the roasted veggies to make a salad bowl (see Buddha Bowls) on occasion and enjoy the hot-and-cold effect of this meal.

- 1 medium sweet, russet, or white sweet potato, peeled and cut into 1- to 2-inch cubes
- 1 small red onion, cut into 1-inch cubes (see notes)
- 1 small celery root, cut into 1- to 2-inch cubes
- 1 small butternut squash, peeled and cut into 1- to 2-inch cubes
- 1 to 2 tablespoons olive, coconut, or avocado oil
- 1 teaspoon dried herbs (garlic and herb, basil, oregano, or nutritional yeast)

Preheat the oven to 375°F.

Put all your cut-up vegetables on a parchment-lined baking sheet or two. Coat the vegetables with the oil (pump sprays work well too) and mix well with your hands to evenly distribute the oil. Don't crowd them, as then they could steam instead of roast. Sprinkle the vegetables with your favorite dried herbs and salt and pepper to taste.

Put the trays in the oven and roast for 20 minutes, check, flip any smaller vegetables, if needed. Cook an additional 20 minutes if they are not yet tender. Some smaller vegetables will cook faster, so you can check for doneness by piercing the veggies with a fork. The fork should go in easily, and the vegetables will have lightly browned, crispy edges as they start to caramelize.

NOTES: Serving size can be adapted depending on what you have on hand. Using up vegetables so they are not wasted is always encouraged.

If onions cause any discomfort, omit as needed.

For a healthy dose of omega-3s and protein, in addition to other nutrients, top roasted vegetables with a serving of hemp hearts.

COLLARD GREEN WRAPS WITH ORANGE-TAHINI HERB SAUCE
MAKES 2 TO 3 WRAPS

Using collard greens in place of tortillas is a home run in the superfoods category. High levels of vitamin K help your body absorb calcium and could, in turn, strengthen your bones. They also have a decent amount of protein, folate, and iron.

To better digest the greens in Reset, we blanch them. This is great for meal prep as well. Once you blanch the greens, store them in the fridge, separated by paper towels, to use later in the week. After Reset, try adding refried beans, hummus, or mashed beans for a hearty dose of calcium, protein, folate, fiber, and antioxidants.

WRAPS:

- 6 to 8 collard greens
- 1 large sweet potato, roasted, peeled, and sliced
- 1 roasted red bell pepper, peeled and sliced into strips (see notes)
- Handful of sprouted greens (alfalfa, pea shoots, arugula)
- 1 avocado, sliced
- ¼ cup cooked quinoa

ORANGE-TAHINI HERB SAUCE:

- 2 tablespoons tahini
- ¼ cup fresh-squeezed orange juice
- ¼ teaspoon orange zest
- ¼ cup hot water
- 1 teaspoon pesto (see notes)

Wash the greens and cut off the thick stem at the base of each leaf. Use a small knife to trim the thick spine down the middle of the leaf. You can also cut the stem out entirely if it's too thick. If you cut the stem out, you will be left with half a leaf, which makes it much easier to roll.

Bring 1 cup of salted water to a boil. Add one leaf and gently move it around with a wooden spoon. The leaf will blanch in about 45 seconds. Remove it and submerge it in a bowl of ice water for 10 seconds. Repeat with the remaining leaves.

Lay out the leaves separately and let air-dry for a couple of minutes. You can also blot excess water with a paper towel.

To make the Orange-Tahini Herb Sauce, put all the sauce ingredients in a high-speed blender or blender cup and blend until smooth. You can double the recipe and use the extra sauce in a salad or as a dipping sauce for roasted vegetables. This will keep for a week in the refrigerator.

Create 2 to 3 circles with the leaves (or leaf halves), overlapping them slightly to prevent holes. Fill each circle with an equal amount of the filling ingredients, starting with the sauce, unless you prefer to use it as a dipping sauce. Make sure your ingredients are toward the bottom of the circle of leaves. Fold over the edges and roll it up like a burrito.

Slice each roll in half and serve. Extras will hold up well in the refrigerator for 2 days.

NOTES: A paper towel works well to remove the charred skin from the roasted red bell pepper.

Mixed Herb Pesto or Tarragon Pesto would bring this over the moon with flavor. If you want to use a store-bought pesto, look for vegan types with no nuts.

BAKED GREEN PEA FALAFEL WITH ORANGE-TAHINI HERB SAUCE
MAKES ABOUT 2 DOZEN FALAFEL

These are not your typical falafel, but by taking the traditional concept and reinventing it, these tasty bites are now fitting for the Reset 90/10 program. Green peas are highly nutritious and a rich source of plant-based protein. These falafel are easy to make and can be frozen once cooked to make mealtime easier. The possibilities are endless: snacks, an appetizer, filling for a collard green wrap, a salad topper, or dinner with a baked potato.

- 2 tablespoons olive, coconut, or avocado oil
- ¼ cup ground flaxseed
- ¼ cup hemp hearts
- 1 tablespoon lemon juice
- 1 cup cooked white rice or whole-grain buckwheat (see notes)
- 2 cups frozen or fresh peas, blanched
- 2 cups sautéed or steamed baby greens, chopped (spinach, kale, Swiss chard, or a combination)
- 1 (14-ounce) jar or can artichokes or artichoke hearts, rinsed and chopped
- 1 teaspoon ground cumin
- 1 teaspoon ground tarragon or ¼ cup fresh tarragon
- ½ teaspoon dried herb blend (I use a dried vegetable blend from The Dandelion Kitchen)
- ½ teaspoon pepper
- ½ teaspoon sea salt
- ½ cup Orange-Tahini Herb Sauce (see Collard Green Wraps)

Preheat the oven to 400°F. Line a baking sheet with parchment paper and lightly coat with the oil (pump sprays work well too).

In a large bowl, combine the flaxseed, hemp hearts, and lemon juice and let sit for 5 minutes. Add the cooked rice, peas, baby greens, artichokes, cumin, tarragon, herb blend, pepper, and salt and mix well. Put the mixture in a food processer and process on high for about 30 seconds, making sure all the ingredients are well combined. Transfer the mixture back to the bowl. Scoop out 1-inch balls and space them evenly on the prepared baking sheet. Press each down gently to form oval patties.

Bake in the oven for 20 minutes. Flip and bake for an additional 20 minutes. They should be golden brown and crispy. Serve with the sauce.

NOTES: After Reset, you can try this with brown rice instead.

Also after Reset, consider adding ½ teaspoon chili powder if spice does not upset your stomach or give you reflux.

MASHED TURNIPS, CELERY ROOT, AND POTATOES
MAKES 2 SERVINGS

This combination of root vegetables is a keeper—add it to your weekly rotation. Celery root is an antioxidant-rich vegetable high in bone-building vitamins and minerals. It is also gut healthy and a rich source of fiber. Same for turnips, but did you know that they contain protein and omega-3 fatty acids in addition to all the other benefits? The potato—full of antioxidants and beneficial nutrients—ties these wonderful flavors together and helps deliver a consistency like a bowl of comforting and creamy mashed potatoes.

- 1 large or 2 medium turnips
- 1 celery root
- 2 small Yukon Gold potatoes
- 3 cloves Roasted Garlic (optional)
- ¼ cup nondairy milk
- ¼ to ½ cup vegetable broth
- Celery salt (optional)
- Fresh rosemary, charred and chopped, or dried herbs (optional, see note)

Peel your turnips, celery root, and potatoes. Roughly cut them into 2- to 3-inch pieces and put them in a large pot of salted water. Bring the pot to a boil over high heat, and simmer for 12 to 15 minutes or until a fork glides easily through the vegetables.

Drain the vegetables, then put them back in the pot over low heat for about a minute to evaporate any remaining water. Add the garlic, milk, and ¼ cup vegetable broth. With a hand masher or immersion blender, blend the mixture. I recommend hand mashing first and then using the immersion blender to create a creamy result. If it's too thick, add more vegetable broth and blend again.

Season with celery salt or any combination of spices that suits your taste, salt, and pepper.

NOTE: Char the rosemary with a torch or over a stove flame. Just enough to make it crackle and turn brown. This will add a nice smoky flavor and keep the rosemary from overpowering the mash.

ROASTED SWEET POTATO FRIED RICE
MAKES 4 SERVINGS

This simple go-to meal is a huge time-saver with minimal prep involved when you use riced sweet potatoes from the freezer section. After Reset, adding in frozen riced cauliflower or broccoli is highly encouraged to reap the benefits of these sulfur-rich vegetables. I have included a small amount of rice at times, along with roasted potatoes, as all the different textures and tastes are delicious and full of fiber-rich and gut-friendly nutrients.

- 2 tablespoons olive, coconut, or avocado oil
- 2 (12-ounce) bags of frozen riced sweet potatoes (see note)
- 2 potatoes, any type, diced (optional)
- 2 tablespoons dried herbs of choice (garlic and herb blend, vegetable blend, chimichurri blend)
- ½ cup cooked white rice or quinoa (optional)
- 1 cup frozen peas and carrots blend, blanched
- 1 (8-ounce) can water chestnuts, drained and roughly chopped (optional)
- 1 bunch asparagus, blanched and diced (optional)
- 1 medium avocado, diced
- 3 scallions or chives, diced
- ¼ cup fresh cilantro, chopped
- 1 cup Chef Lisa DeNiear's Cilantro-Lime Sauce (optional)

Preheat the oven to 375°F. Line a large baking sheet with parchment paper and lightly coat it with the oil (pump sprays work well too).

Place the riced sweet potato and potatoes (if using) on the baking sheet and spread them out evenly. Sprinkle the dried herbs over the top and place in the oven.

Roast for 15 minutes, stir, and smooth out again. Roast for another 25 minutes. Remove from the oven and mix in the rice (if using), peas and carrots, water chestnuts, and asparagus. Season with salt and pepper to taste.

Serve with the avocado, scallions, and cilantro. Dress with cilantro-lime sauce (if using) or coconut aminos.

NOTE: If you can't find frozen riced sweet potatoes, using fresh is also an option. Just rice the raw sweet potatoes in a food processor. The cooking time in the oven may be shorter if you're using fresh.

BAKED POTATO FRIES OR CHIPS
MAKES 4 SERVINGS

Baking potatoes as fries or chips is a fun way to snack or incorporate potatoes into meals. Leftovers can be used for lunch or dinner the next day.

+ 2 tablespoons olive, coconut, or avocado oil
+ 6 small or 4 medium russet, sweet, Japanese white, or purple potatoes (see notes)
+ 2 tablespoons dried herb blend (garlic and herb or lemon pepper, see notes)

Preheat the oven to 375°F. Line a baking sheet with parchment paper and lightly coat it with the oil (pump sprays work well too).

Peel and slice the potatoes into ½-inch wedges or ¼-inch round chips. Your slices do not have to be perfect.

Spread the potatoes out on the baking sheet; use two if needed. Season with dried herbs and salt and pepper.

For wedges, bake for 20 minutes, flip, and bake for another 20 minutes.

For chips, bake for 20 minutes, flip, and bake for another 10 to 15 minutes.

For either version, the potatoes should look golden brown and be easily pierced with a fork when done.

NOTES: When it comes to potatoes, mix it up and benefit from the many nutrients provided by different varieties. They all have different tastes and textures when baked. You won't be sorry!

For the seasoning, any type of savory blend of herbs using rosemary, thyme, oregano, sage, or parsley will do.

SIMPLY MASHED
MAKES ABOUT 4 SERVINGS

It's called "Simply Mashed" because this is a simple recipe with many uses. Try to make these nutritious, filling vegetables a staple in your home, as the resistant starch is so beneficial to your digestive tract. This recipe works with any root vegetable. It's versatile and perfect as a side, quick pick-me-up, or filling for a veggie bowl.

- ½ teaspoon salt
- 6 medium Yukon Gold potatoes, peeled and cut into rough medium-large chunks
- 1 sweet potato, peeled and cut into medium-large chunks (see note)
- 4 parsnips or carrots, peeled and cut into medium-large chunks
- 4 cloves Roasted Garlic (optional)
- ½ cup vegetable broth
- 1 tablespoon fresh herbs, chopped (thyme, rosemary, or chives), or 1 teaspoon dried herbs of choice

Bring a pot of water (enough to cover the vegetables) and ½ teaspoon salt to a boil, add the Yukon Gold potatoes, sweet potato, and parsnips and simmer for 25 to 30 minutes or until the vegetables are tender. A fork should effortlessly pierce your vegetables when done.

Drain the vegetables, then put them back in the pot over low heat for about a minute to evaporate any remaining water.

Mash the vegetables with a potato masher. Add the roasted garlic (if using), broth, and herbs and incorporate with the masher. Use an immersion blender if you would like to achieve a creamier consistency. Add salt and pepper to taste. Depending on the vegetables you use, additional broth may be needed if it seems too dry.

NOTE: Make this recipe your own. Instead of the sweet potato, try any other root vegetable you might have, such as butternut squash, pumpkin, acorn squash, kabocha squash, or celery root.

ENGLISH METHOD OF ROASTING POTATOES AND CARROTS
MAKES 4 SERVINGS

This is my favorite way to enjoy potatoes—it delivers a delicate and smooth taste. The potatoes and carrots are parboiled and then baked, resulting in a delicious golden crunchy exterior and creamy interior.

- 1 teaspoon salt
- 6 medium or 8 small Yukon Gold or 4 medium russet potatoes, peeled and cut into 2-inch pieces
- 6 medium carrots, peeled and cut into 2-inch pieces
- ¼ cup olive, coconut, or avocado oil

Preheat the oven to 375°F. Line a baking sheet with parchment paper.

Bring a pot of water (enough to cover the vegetables) and 1 teaspoon salt to a boil. Add the potatoes and carrots and boil for 8 minutes. Fully drain the vegetables in a colander, add them back to the pot, and shake the pot for about 30 seconds to roughen them up. Add the oil and shake gently to evenly coat the vegetables. Transfer them to the baking sheet and roast for 20 minutes. Flip the vegetables and roast for an additional 10 minutes. They should be golden brown and crunchy looking when done. Season with salt and pepper to taste.

CHERRY TOMATO PASTA
MAKES 2 SERVINGS

Do you have a bowl of cherry or plum tomatoes just staring at you? Turning produce into an effortlessly elegant meal is incredibly simple. Just turn

on the oven! With some plant-based pasta and fresh basil, this can be the most straightforward yet satisfying use of what's in your pantry. Adding some olives or capers seals the deal; both are rich in antioxidants, healthy fat, and vitamin E, all while helping combat inflammation.

- 2 pints cherry tomatoes
- ¼ cup olive, coconut, or avocado oil
- 6 stalks asparagus, cut into 2-inch pieces
- 2 shallots, thinly sliced
- 4 ounces buckwheat or rice-based pasta
- 1 tablespoon capers
- 6 olives
- ½ teaspoon lemon zest, or ¼ cup lemon juice
- ¼ cup vegetable broth
- ½ cup fresh basil
- Nutritional yeast (optional)

Preheat the oven to 375°F. Line a roasting pan with parchment paper.

Put the oil and tomatoes in a large bowl. Stir to coat the tomatoes with the oil, then put them in the prepared roasting pan. Roast for 10 minutes and then remove the pan from the oven. Add the shallots and asparagus and return the pan to the oven, roasting for an additional 20 minutes. The tomatoes will be slightly browned and the asparagus al dente.

While the vegetables are roasting, cook your pasta in salted water according to the package directions. Remove from the heat when al dente and drain thoroughly. If using buckwheat pasta, I recommend a quick hot water rinse, as it can get quite starchy.

When the vegetables are done, put the pasta back into the pot along with the capers, olives, lemon zest, and vegetable broth. Put the pot on the stovetop over medium heat. Add the roasted tomatoes, asparagus, and shallots and gently fold everything together. Stir in the fresh basil, remove from the heat, and serve. Add salt and pepper to taste to make all the flavors pop. Garnish with nutritional yeast.

BAKED POTATOES
MAKES 2 SERVINGS

*Turning a baked potato into lunch or dinner is a simple way to effi-
ciently get good nutrients when life is chaotic. Remember—during the
Reset phase, do not eat the skin. Although extremely nutritious, digesting potato skin is tough on the gut.*

- 2 russet or sweet potatoes

TOPPINGS TO TRY:

- Pesto and sliced avocado
- Salsa, olives, sliced avocado, and hempseeds
- Sautéed greens, artichokes, and nutritional yeast
- Sautéed greens, asparagus, and mushrooms

Preheat the oven to 425°F. Line a baking sheet with foil or parchment
paper.

Scrub the potatoes thoroughly. Prick each several times with a fork
to allow steam to release during the cooking process. Lay the potatoes
on the prepared baking sheet and put it in the oven. Bake for 50 to 60
minutes, flipping the potatoes every 20 minutes or so and checking for
doneness by piercing them with a fork. The potatoes are done when the
skins are dry and the insides are completely soft.

ROASTED FROZEN VEGETABLES
YIELD VARIES

*Vegetables straight from the freezer into your oven are a wonderful
replacement for fresh when you need dinner in a pinch. Most vegetables are frozen at their peak of ripeness and are tasty when roasted.
Cooking times may vary with certain smaller vegetables like green
beans and asparagus spears. Make that judgment call after the first
15 minutes in the oven.*

- 1 bag frozen vegetables of choice
- 2 tablespoons olive, coconut, or avocado oil
- 1 to 2 tablespoons dried herb blend of choice
- Fresh herbs, chopped (optional)

Preheat the oven to 375°F. Line a baking sheet with parchment paper.

Put your frozen vegetables in a bowl and lightly coat them with the oil (pump sprays work well too). Spread the vegetables out in a single layer on the prepared baking sheet and sprinkle them with dried herbs.

Depending on the size and type of the vegetables, cooking times may vary. Check the vegetables after 15 minutes and flip if they are starting to brown. Add fresh herbs (if using), and cook for an additional 10 to 15 minutes. Season with salt and pepper.

Using frozen vegetables doesn't have to be a scary thought with the following tips to save time and get the most out of this convenience food. First, they don't require much cooking time, because they are parcooked, so you are basically just reheating them. Steaming or blanching frozen vegetables is the quickest, most effective stovetop method. Boiling often results in overcooked, mushy vegetables that are unappealing.

- If you are making pasta, consider adding something like green beans, broccoli, or peas to the pasta pot for the last minute of cook time, then drain the added vegetables along with the pasta. From there, add your favorite sauce or pesto.
- Frozen vegetables are a convenient way to add greens like frozen spinach, kale, or cauliflower to a smoothie (see Salted Chocolate Date Smoothie with a Twist). No thawing required!
- Frozen vegetables are a great addition to soups, stews, and casserole-type dishes. When a meal has a combination of ingredients, there is no need to

worry about texture. Ingredients in dishes like these are almost foolproof, and that allows for fun and creative adventures in the kitchen.

- Frozen vegetables may require a little more seasoning than fresh. There is an abundance of fresh herbs at your supermarket worth experimenting with. If you are lucky enough to grow your own, I recommend adding fresh herbs to a dish close to the end of or after cooking. Softer herbs like fresh basil, oregano, mint, and parsley are a wonderful last-minute enhancement to cooked vegetables. Roasting other fresh herbs like rosemary, thyme, marjoram, and sage along with the vegetables can open up their flavors and aromas.
- Dried herbs can also make an unforgettable experience at mealtime. Take an ordinary frozen veggie and experiment with adding dried herbs to find what works for you. See the following list and don't be afraid to spice it up with herbs, spices, and acids.

Herb Combinations to Try

- Asparagus: basil, dill, garlic, lemon
- Beans: basil, garlic, lemon, onion
- Beets: basil, cilantro, dill, lemon, mint, orange, tarragon
- Broccoli: basil, lemon, oregano
- Brussels sprouts: garlic, parsley, rosemary
- Carrots: cumin, dill, ginger, sage, tarragon
- Potatoes (sweet): cinnamon, cumin, garlic, paprika
- Potatoes (white): basil, cumin, chili powder, garlic, rosemary, sage; lemon is always a wonderful enhancement to roasted potatoes
- Squash (summer): basil, parsley, oregano
- Squash (winter): basil, thyme, rosemary
- Spinach: basil, dill, garlic, lemon

ROASTED ACORN SQUASH
MAKES 2 SERVINGS

Roasting an acorn squash is an efficient way to change things up a bit and reap the benefits of this slightly sweet, antioxidant-rich food. Cutting the squash in half may require a little elbow grease and a good knife, but it's worth the effort. Plus, the shell serves as a bowl that you can stuff with almost anything, like leftover veggies and grains.

Get creative with your leftover squash too! Chunks can grace a salad the next day. It can become a layer in a veggie lasagna or quesadilla after Reset. It can even be added to an impromptu pureed soup. The peel is edible as well, but avoid the peel in Reset for optimal digestive perks.

- 2 tablespoons olive, coconut, or avocado oil
- 1 acorn squash (see note)
- 1 teaspoon dried herb blend of choice (basil, parsley, oregano)
- 2 cloves Roasted Garlic (optional)
- Olive oil (optional)
- Lemon juice (optional)

Preheat the oven to 375°F. Line a baking sheet with parchment paper and lightly coat it with the oil (pump sprays work well too).

To cut the squash, start on one side of the stem and cut straight through until the knife hits the hollow middle, then out through the other side and down to the bottom of the squash.

Pull apart the halves, remove the seeds, and trim the stem (optional). After Reset, you can save the seeds to roast and eat; they make a great snack or addition to a salad—yum!

Season the halves with your favorite dried herbs and roasted garlic (if using). Place the halves cut side down on the prepared baking sheet.

Roast for 40 to 50 minutes. A knife should easily slide through the skin and into the flesh when it is done. Flip the squash carefully to release the steam after cooking. Add a drizzle of good olive oil or lemon juice (if using). These are a nice finish and complement this delicious vegetable. Season with salt and pepper to taste.

NOTE: Other varieties of winter squash, like butternut, kabocha, or pumpkin, also work well in this recipe.

STEAMED VEGETABLES
MAKES 2 SERVINGS

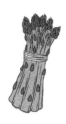

Steaming is one of the quickest and easiest ways to get vegetables on your plate. The trick to steaming multiple fresh vegetables is to cut them up into similar-sized pieces. Some vegetables are steamed in 3 minutes, and some take a little longer. With the following guide, you'll be steaming any and every vegetable.

- 2 carrots, peeled and cut on the bias into ½-inch pieces
- 4 spears of asparagus, cut into 2-inch pieces
- 1 medium zucchini, cut into 1-inch rounds
- Lemon or lime juice (optional)
- A drizzle of olive oil (optional)
- Dried herb blend of choice (optional)

Fill a large pot with a steamer basket with about 1 inch of water. The water should be right under the basket without touching it. Bring the water to a boil over high heat, then put the vegetables in the steamer basket. You will get the best results when the thickest vegetables (carrots in this recipe) are on the bottom and the smallest ones are on top.

Cover the pot and simmer. Check the vegetables after the allotted time (see the chart) to see if a knife can easily slide through the thickest part. Vegetables are done when they are tender but still have a slight crunch.

Drizzle with fresh lemon or lime juice and a dash of olive oil and season with herbs or salt and pepper.

NOTE: Save the leftover water for a vegetable stock. Stocks are a wonderful way to utilize often-tossed leftover vegetables and scraps.

Vegetable Cooking Time Guide

Artichokes	20 to 30 minutes depending on size
Asparagus, pieces	4 to 5 minutes
Asparagus, whole	7 to 8 minutes
Beets, whole and unpeeled	35 to 50 minutes
Broccoli or cauliflower florets	5 to 7 minutes
Brussels sprouts, trimmed and whole	8 to 15 minutes
Brussels sprouts, trimmed and halved	6 to 8 minutes
Cabbage wedges	6 to 10 minutes
Carrots	10 to 12 minutes
Green beans	3 to 5 minutes
Jerusalem artichokes (sunchokes), peeled and scrubbed	5 to 8 minutes
Kale, collard, and other hearty greens	8 to 10 minutes
Okra	6 to 8 minutes
Onions	8 to 12 minutes
Parsnips	10 to 12 minutes
Peas	3 minutes
Peas and carrots	3 to 4 minutes
Potatoes	8 to 12 minutes
Spinach, Swiss chard	3 to 4 minutes
Sugar snap peas	5 to 6 minutes
Summer squash, zucchini	5 to 8 minutes
Winter squash, butternut squash, celery root, turnips	8 to 15 minutes

BREAK OUT THE SPIRALIZER
YIELD VARIES

By far, the most favored way to use a spiralizer has been making zoodles (zucchini noodles)—until now. The possibilities are vast with one of these inexpensive tools and a little imagination and creativity.

- The most obvious way to use a spiralizer is to spiralize zucchini as a replacement for pasta in any dish you like. I like
to make a half-zoodle, half-pasta version so I feel
content with a small portion of pasta when the
mood strikes. A favorite of mine is roasted zucchini spirals with buckwheat noodles and a light
pesto sauce with steamed green beans thrown
in. Other veggies that fit well in pasta dishes are
yellow squash, butternut squash, and radishes.
- Roasting spirals in the oven is easy and can be
done on the fly. Line a baking sheet with parchment paper and lightly coat it with oil (pump
sprays work well too). Add the spirals, dust them with the
dried herbs of your choice, and roast in a 375°F oven for 10
to 15 minutes. You will steam out excess water and get a bit
of golden-brown caramelization. You can even roast spirals
of root vegetables such as beets, carrots, potatoes or turnips
this way, though they will take around 20 to 30 minutes.

  You'll be tempted to devour these right from the oven,
  but consider layering the finished product on top of a
  simple salad with olives and one of the recipes from the
  Condiments, Sauces, Dips, and Spreads section for a tasty,
  satisfying lunch or dinner option.
- Reinvent some of your favorite recipes! Spiralized vegetables can be layered into casserole-type dishes, soups,
lasagnas, salads, and even ramen or other noodle bowls
(replacing pasta noodles).

CREAM OF BUCKWHEAT BLUEBERRY CEREAL
MAKES 2 SERVINGS

*How about breakfast for lunch or dinner? This gluten-free alternative to
oats may be what you are looking for on those cool fall or winter days.
I've taken buckwheat cereal a step further and added fresh and frozen
fruit with tasty results. If you are not a fan of blueberries, substitute*

apples (see notes). Also consider a serving of ground hempseed or ground flaxseed for a boost of protein, iron, and omegas.

- 3 cups water or nondairy milk (I use half water, half oat milk)
- ½ teaspoon salt
- ½ cup Cream of Buckwheat cereal
- 1 cup frozen blueberries
- 1 mashed banana
- Honey or maple syrup (optional)

In a medium saucepan, bring the water and salt to a boil. Stir in the Cream of Buckwheat cereal and then the blueberries and banana.

Reduce the heat to low and simmer for about 10 minutes, stirring constantly. If you notice it getting too thick, add a little extra water to thin it out. Think about how you like your oatmeal and aim for a similar consistency. Finish with a touch of honey (if using).

NOTES: Not a fan of blueberries? Make the cereal according to the directions and add 1 cup fresh or store-bought applesauce plus ½ teaspoon cinnamon to the pot in place of the blueberries.

If you are eating this in the morning, consider other toppings, such as sliced fresh banana or a couple of fresh blueberries, for a picture-perfect breakfast.

BUCKWHEAT PANCAKES
MAKES ABOUT 20 PANCAKES (SEE NOTES)

If you're missing breakfast foods during Reset, try these pancakes for lunch or dinner. Ground flax is a great way to get plant-based protein: it is rich in omega-3s, high in fiber, and great for reducing cholesterol and lowering blood pressure. This tasty and filling nutrient-dense alternative to your typical pancake is a keeper.

- 3 tablespoons ground flaxseed
- ¼ cup water
- 2 cups buckwheat flour

- 1 teaspoon baking powder
- 1 teaspoon baking soda
- ½ teaspoon salt
- 1 teaspoon Pumpkin Pie Spice
- 2 cups nondairy milk
- ½ cup unsweetened applesauce, plus more for serving (optional)
- 2 mashed bananas
- 1 cup frozen blueberries (see notes)
- Olive, coconut, or avocado oil
- Maple syrup (optional)
- 1 cup Fresh or Frozen Fruit Sauce (optional)

In a medium bowl, create the flax egg by combining the flaxseed and water and letting it sit for 5 minutes.

While you are waiting, in a large bowl, combine the buckwheat flour, baking powder, baking soda, salt, and Pumpkin Pie Spice.

After your flax egg is set, add the nondairy milk, applesauce, and banana (it's okay if it's a bit lumpy) to the medium bowl and stir. Fold in the frozen blueberries. Add the wet ingredients to the dry and stir until well combined. Let the batter sit for 5 minutes.

Grease a skillet with the oil (pump sprays work too) and heat it over medium heat. Add ¼-cup dollops of the prepared batter to the skillet. Cook over medium to medium-high heat, wait for the pancakes to bubble—4 to 5 minutes—then flip. The pancakes are done when both sides are browned and set.

Serve hot with maple syrup, more unsweetened applesauce, or Fresh or Frozen Fruit Sauce, whatever you like.

NOTES: This is a big recipe, but you can freeze half and be super prepared for snacks or mealtime in the following weeks.

If using frozen blueberries, let them sit for several minutes as they will release some moisture. You can also use any fresh fruit of your choice, but you might end up needing a little more milk if the batter is too thick.

SALADS

SIMPLE SALAD
MAKES 2 SERVINGS

Simple salads are highly encouraged throughout Reset, as the greens are a major player in proper elimination. Consider soft lettuces, add-in options, and fresh herbs. Herbs don't last long, so if you need to use them up, toss them on your salad. There are too many remarkable healing properties associated with fresh herbs to let them go to waste. Build your salad with these four easy steps.

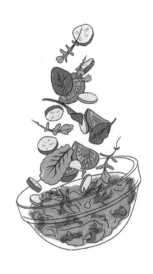

Choose about 2 cups of the following greens: Bibb, Boston, butter, red leaf, and romaine lettuces. Chop roughly into bite-size pieces and divide between two bowls.

Add one or a combination of the following: 1 cup sliced and peeled cucumber and/or diced tomato, 1 diced avocado, 1 teaspoon capers, 10 whole olives. Divide between two bowls.

Add about 1 tablespoon roughly chopped herbs of your choice divided between bowls. Delicious complementary herbs include basil, cilantro, chives, dill, lemon balm, parsley, and mint.

Add your choice of vinaigrette or dressing to each bowl and mix everything together.

BUCKWHEAT AND ROASTED VEGETABLE TABBOULEH SALAD
MAKES 4 TO 5 SERVINGS

Whole-grain buckwheat is a good source of fiber and protein and includes all essential amino acids. Amino acids help build muscle and regulate immune function and our precious hormones. The hulled buckwheat is like barley, with a similar nutty and hearty flavor, but it's void of gluten for those with sensitivities. Hulled buckwheat is also a great addition to a soup, stew, or porridge-type dish.

I love this salad at room temperature because I find the flavors really pop when they are not as cold. If you are having this for dinner during the Reset phase, add a couple of olives or diced avocado for a balanced dinner option. Extras make a great lunch the next day.

- 1 cup cooked hulled buckwheat (see notes)
- ½ butternut squash, diced and roasted (about 1½ cups, see notes)
- 3 yellow beets, peeled, roasted, and diced (see notes)
- 4 stalks asparagus, blanched and roughly chopped (optional)
- ½ cup fresh parsley, finely chopped

SAUCE:

- ⅓ cup lemon juice
- 3 scallions, chopped
- ¼ cup olive oil
- 2 tablespoons fresh tarragon, chopped
- 1 tablespoon lemon zest
- 1 tablespoon fresh mint, chopped
- 1 tablespoon maple syrup

Prepare the sauce in a small bowl by gently whisking together all the ingredients.

In a large bowl, combine the cooked buckwheat, squash, beets, asparagus (if using), and parsley. Fold the sauce into the buckwheat mixture. Serve immediately. Season with salt and pepper to taste.

NOTES: When shopping for hulled buckwheat, look for packaging that says "organic hulled whole grain." I recommend rinsing the buckwheat after it is cooked, as it sometimes becomes very starchy.

Roast butternut squash and beets as follows: Preheat the oven to 375°F. Place all your cut-up vegetables on a parchment-lined baking sheet or two. Coat the vegetables with oil (pump sprays work well too) and mix well with your hands to evenly distribute the oil. Don't crowd the veggies, as then they could steam instead of roast. Sprinkle the vegetables with your favorite dried herbs. Put the trays in the oven and roast for 20 minutes, check, and flip any smaller vegetables, if needed. You may want to remove the asparagus at this point depending on its thickness. Roast for an additional 20 minutes if they are not yet tender. Some smaller vegetables will cook faster, so you can check by piercing the veggies with a fork. The fork should go in easily, and the vegetables will have lightly browned, crispy edges as they start to caramelize.

RAW PAD THAI NOODLE SALAD
MAKES 2 SERVINGS

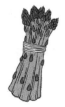

This is such a yummy salad that you can build up in so many ways after the Reset phase. You can also find prepackaged fresh or frozen spiralized vegetables in most supermarkets for a quicker version.

- 2 small or 1 large green zucchini, spiralized (see notes)
- 1 yellow squash, spiralized
- 4 stalks asparagus, blanched and diced
- ½ cup peas and carrots, blanched (frozen bags come in handy here)
- 1 cup microgreens (radish, beets, arugula, watercress, pea shoots)
- Avocado slices
- 2 scallions, chopped
- Handful of fresh cilantro, chopped
- Lime wedges

TAHINI SAUCE (SEE NOTES):

- 2 tablespoons tahini
- 2 tablespoons coconut aminos
- 2 tablespoons coconut vinegar
- 2 tablespoons water
- 1 tablespoon lime juice
- 1 tablespoon maple syrup, or 1 Medjool date, pitted (see notes)
- Handful of fresh cilantro
- 1 teaspoon fresh ginger, grated
- ½ teaspoon cayenne or red chili flakes (optional)

To make the tahini sauce, put all the sauce ingredients in a high-speed blender and blend until thick and smooth. You may need to add a bit more water if the consistency is extremely thick. The result should be thick but creamy—something that will stick to a spoon. This is a good consistency for sticking to the noodles. Season with salt and pepper.

Put the zucchini and squash zoodles, asparagus, and peas and carrots into a large bowl and mix together. If you are not making both servings, store the raw veggies separate from the dressing. They will keep for 3 days.

When you are ready to serve, add 1 tablespoon of tahini sauce for each serving to the zoodle mixture. Fold the sauce into the vegetables. To serve, split the microgreens and veggie mixture between the bowls, then top with avocado, scallions, cilantro, and a squeeze of fresh lime juice. Season with salt and pepper to taste.

NOTES: The tahini sauce is easy to make a double batch of and will keep in the refrigerator for 10 days.

If your date is not very soft, soak it in a small bowl of warm water for about 10 minutes.

If using fresh squash, spiralize, then lay the spirals flat on a tray lined with paper towels. Lightly salt the zoodles and let them sweat for 5 to 10 minutes. Use the paper towels to blot excess moisture. Now you will have super dry zoodles that are extra crunchy and won't compromise this delicious salad with excess water. You can also use 12-ounce prepackaged frozen zoodles, which you'll need to defrost. I recommend laying them on a kitchen towel or paper towels as they're defrosting because they may get very wet. Typical frozen packages yield 4 servings, so for this recipe, use only half a 12-ounce package.

After Reset, you can consider other optional add-ins, like chopped red or green cabbage, sprouts, and roasted pumpkin seeds.

BUDDHA BOWLS
YIELD VARIES

A Buddha bowl is any combination of grains, veggies, protein, dressing, and garnishes served in a bowl. Becoming creative with this one-dish meal is a fun way to use up leftover vegetables, grains, and dressings (sauces). In Reset, remember we are excluding protein sources like beans and legumes. But there is protein in vegetables such as potatoes, asparagus, peas, buckwheat, tahini, and quinoa—the list goes on! Get creative to build a balanced bowl.

After Reset, adding in beans, lentils, broccoli, brussels sprouts, nuts, and seeds will make for a quick mealtime favorite. Here are a couple of options to get you started, though the combinations are endless.

Buddha Bowls Sample Combinations

Grain/Base	Vegetables/ Greens	Protein	Dressing	Garnishes
Quinoa	Roasted vegetables	Baked Green Pea Falafel	Chef Lisa DeNiear's Cilantro-Lime Sauce	Chopped cilantro and scallions
Baked Potato Fries	Steamed asparagus and peas	Sliced avocado or 2 tablespoons ground flaxseed	Tahini Sauce	Quick Pickled Radish, chopped cilantro
Whole-grain buckwheat	Salad greens, peeled cucumber, tomatoes	Hemp hearts	Whipped Tahini Sauce	Beet Salsa and chopped parsley and dill
Simply Mashed	Roasted eggplant and peppers	Nutritional yeast	Mixed Herb Pesto	Diced avocado
Quinoa	Sautéed spinach and diced sweet potato	Steamed mung bean sprouts	Green Goddess Vinaigrette	Kalamata olives
White rice	Salad greens, roasted butternut squash	Yuzu Pea Puree	Simple Salad Vinaigrette	Diced avocado and chopped tarragon
Brown rice (after Reset)	Steamed broccoli (after Reset)	Vegetarian Lentil Meatballs (after Reset)	Sun-Dried Tomato Spread (after Reset)	Toasted pumpkin seeds (after Reset) and chopped oregano and parsley

SOUPS

TOMATO, FENNEL, AND SWEET POTATO SOUP
MAKES 3 TO 4 SERVINGS

Fennel is a supportive vegetable that aids in digestive processes by reducing inflammation and bad bacteria and feeding good bacteria with prebiotic-rich properties. Fennel also stimulates the secretion of vital digestive enzymes. This combination is a keeper.

- 2 tablespoons olive, coconut, or avocado oil
- 2 large or 4 small fennel bulbs, roughly chopped
- 2 large leeks, trimmed, cleaned, and roughly chopped (tender parts only, discard the tougher outer green part)
- 1 large or 2 small sweet potatoes, peeled and cut into rough ½-inch pieces
- 5 tomatoes, chopped, or 1 (28-ounce) can tomatoes
- 5 cups vegetable broth
- Bouquet garni of fresh thyme, parsley, bay leaf, and rosemary

In a large soup pot, combine the oil, fennel, leeks, and sweet potatoes. Sauté over high heat for several minutes. Add the tomatoes, broth, and bouquet garni. Bring the soup to a boil, then let simmer for 40 minutes.

Remove the bouquet garni and use an immersion blender to blend the soup until smooth. You can also blend the soup in small batches in a high-speed blender once it has slightly cooled.

Season with salt and pepper to taste and serve hot.

Bouquet Garni

Bouquet garni is a French term that translates to "garnished bouquet." It is used mainly to add flavor and depth to soups, stews, and beans— really anything that simmers. All you need is some kitchen twine, herbs, and your imagination. A typical bouquet includes a few sprigs each of parsley and thyme and several bay leaves. Leek leaves can be wrapped around the herbs and secured with butcher's string, or you can create a cheesecloth bundle and add in spices like peppercorn. Remember to experiment!

CELERY ROOT, ASPARAGUS, AND TURNIP SOUP
MAKES 6 SERVINGS

Picking the most-healing ingredients for the Reset stage is done with much consideration. This soup gets high marks because celery root is high in antioxidants, complex B vitamins, vitamins C and K, and much-needed minerals. Turnip is just as impressive with high fiber, folate, iron, calcium, and protein. In addition, spotlighting one of my favorite superfoods, asparagus just seems to make sense in this recipe. All three veggies merge in this delicious puree to provide an anti-inflammatory and gut-friendly soup you will make time and time again.

- 2 tablespoons olive, coconut, or avocado oil
- 2 large leeks, trimmed, cleaned, and roughly chopped (tender parts only, discard the tougher outer green part)
- 1 small yellow onion, chopped
- 1 large or 2 small celery roots, peeled and cut into rough cubes
- 1 large or 2 small turnips, peeled and cut into rough cubes

- 1 bunch of asparagus, trim the bottoms and cut into 1-inch lengths (save the tops to roast and use as garnish, optional)
- 1 teaspoon dried tarragon
- 1 teaspoon dried basil
- 1 teaspoon salt
- 1 teaspoon white or black pepper
- 5 to 6 cups vegetable broth
- ½ cup full-fat unsweetened canned coconut milk

Heat the oil in a large pot or Dutch oven over medium heat. Add the leeks and onion and cook, stirring often, for 3 to 4 minutes. Add the celery root, turnips, and asparagus and continue to cook, stirring often, for another 8 minutes. Add in the seasonings and 5 cups of the vegetable broth—enough to just about cover the vegetables so they can simmer. If you feel as though you need more, add the remaining 1 cup broth. Bring to a boil, cover, and simmer over low heat for 30 to 40 minutes.

If you saved the asparagus tips, preheat the oven to 350°F. Put the asparagus tips on a baking sheet lined with parchment paper and roast them for 8 to 10 minutes. Set aside.

Remove the soup from the heat and make sure all the vegetables are tender and cooked through. Add in the coconut milk and blend the soup with an immersion blender until you have a beautiful puree. You can also blend the soup in small batches in a high-speed blender once it has slightly cooled. Season with salt and pepper to taste.

Adding Grains to Soups or Salads

Grains like white rice, quinoa, and whole-grain buckwheat are delicious, filling, and nutritious additions to pureed soups or Buddha Bowls. On those days when you are especially hungry or want to add some depth to your meal, enjoy these grains in moderation—¼ cup per serving. In Reset, we prefer white rice over brown because it is easier to digest and not associated with gastrointestinal issues.

BUTTERNUT SQUASH, FENNEL, AND PEAR SOUP
MAKES 8 TO 9 SERVINGS (SEE NOTES)

This is one of the most delicious, nutritious, and sat-isfying soups in my collection. Coconut milk finishes this soup, making it dairy-free, velvety, and decadent. This soup provides an abundance of health benefits such as immune support and gut healing prebiotic goodness.

- ¼ cup olive, coconut, or avocado oil, divided
- 2 small yellow onions, roughly chopped
- 2 butternut squash, roughly cubed
- 3 fennel bulbs, roughly chopped, and fronds (see notes)
- 3 pears, peeled, halved, and seeded
- 2 large or 4 small white potatoes, peeled and roughly chopped
- 4 carrots, peeled and roughly chopped
- Bouquet garni of fresh rosemary, oregano, and thyme
- 4 to 5 cups vegetable broth
- 1 cup full-fat unsweetened canned coconut milk
- ¼ cup lemon juice
- Fresh thyme
- Salt and white pepper

Preheat the oven to 350°F. Line a baking sheet with parchment paper and lightly coat it with 2 tablespoons of the oil (pump sprays work well too).

Roast the onions, butternut squash, fennel, and pears for 45 minutes. Check after 25 minutes and flip any smaller vegetables.

Put the remaining 2 tablespoons oil, roasted vegetables, potatoes, and carrots in a large stockpot or Dutch oven and cook over medium-high heat for several minutes, stirring occasionally. Add the bouquet garni and 4 cups of the vegetable broth—enough to just about cover the vegetables so they can simmer. If you feel as though you need more, add the remaining 1 cup broth. Bring to a boil, then simmer for 35 minutes.

Remove the bouquet garni. Blend the soup with an immersion blender until creamy. Add in the coconut milk and blend again. At this point, you can adjust the thickness with more broth, if needed. You can also blend the soup in batches in a high-speed blender once it has slightly cooled.

Stir in the lemon juice, thyme, and salt and pepper to taste, garnish with fennel fronds (if using), and serve hot.

NOTES: If you aren't planning a dinner party, any extra soup will freeze beautifully. Freezing soup is convenient and time-saving, but please make sure to cool the soup down properly before it goes into the freezer—use an ice bath to quicken the process. Store the cooled soup in a freezer bag and lay it flat if space is an issue, or consider Souper Cubes (see Resources) for convenient freezer-friendly containers. The safest and best way to thaw soup is to place the container in a warm water bath until fully thawed. Place the thawed soup in a pot and reheat on the stovetop over low heat for best results.

Save the fennel fronds to garnish the dish, use them to make fennel pesto, or add them to your bouquet garni.

GINGER PUMPKIN SOUP
MAKES 6 SERVINGS

This is so incredibly easy to make. Soups are a low-calorie, fiber-rich, nutrient-dense way to fill up any time of the year. Making use of these fall vegetables is a delicious way to incorporate plant-based vitamins, minerals, and disease-fighting antioxidants into your diet.

Ginger's medicinal properties are many. Ginger is great for digestion and reducing inflammation throughout the body. It also aids in lowing blood sugar and cholesterol levels. Roasting the squash prior to adding it to your soup gives the finished product a deeper dimension of flavor, so it's recommended but not necessary.

- 2 to 3 tablespoons olive, coconut, or avocado oil
- 1 cup mirepoix (equal amounts diced carrots, celery, and onion, see notes)

- 1½ tablespoons fresh ginger, grated
- 1 teaspoon ground cumin
- 1 teaspoon ground turmeric
- ½ teaspoon chili powder
- 3 cups butternut squash, chopped (1 small or ½ large, see notes)
- 2 cups fresh pumpkin or other fall squash (acorn, kabocha), diced and roasted, or 1 (15-ounce) can pumpkin puree
- 1 cup dried red lentils (see notes)
- 4 ½ to 5 cups vegetable broth
- Bouquet garni (sage, thyme, parsley, bay leaf, optional)
- Salt and pepper
- ¼ cup full-fat unsweetened canned coconut milk (shake well before opening)
- Roasted pumpkin seeds (optional for after Reset)

Put the oil and the mirepoix in a stockpot and sauté over medium heat for several minutes. Add the ginger, cumin, turmeric, and chili powder. Cook and stir for another two minutes. Add the butternut squash, pumpkin, and lentils. Sauté for 5 minutes over medium-high heat.

Add 4½ cups of the broth. Bring to a boil, then reduce the heat to low-medium. Add the bouquet garni and simmer for at least 40 minutes.

Remove the soup from the stove and let cool for 20 to 30 minutes. Puree with an immersion blender or let cool slightly and blend in batches in a high-speed blender until it's thick and creamy. Stir in the coconut milk. If you find the soup is too thick, thin it out with the last ½ cup of vegetable broth.

Garnish with roasted pumpkin seeds (after Reset), if you like, and serve hot. Season with salt and pepper to taste.

NOTES: You can often find prepared mirepoix in the produce section.

For a richer flavor, I suggest roasting the squash at 375°F for 30 minutes before adding it to the stockpot.

For Reset, omit the lentils and add 1 diced white or sweet potato instead.

THAI ROASTED RED PEPPER SOUP
MAKES 6 SERVINGS

This fiber-filled play on Thai soup is a delicious addition to the Reset recipes. Red peppers are an excellent source of vitamins C, B6, and A. Incorporating something like white basmati rice, quinoa, or buckwheat grains would be a delicious way to add some texture to the soup.

- 2 tablespoons olive, coconut, or avocado oil
- ½ yellow onion, roughly chopped
- 3 parsnips, peeled and diced
- 4 garlic cloves, chopped finely (optional)
- 1 tablespoon fresh ginger, grated
- 1 teaspoon red curry paste or curry powder
- 1 teaspoon ground coriander
- 2 white or orange sweet potatoes, diced
- 5 large red bell peppers, roasted, peeled, and chopped
- 1 (15-ounce can) diced tomatoes or 2 small tomatoes, chopped
- 4 cups vegetable broth
- ½ cup full-fat unsweetened canned coconut milk
- Fresh basil, chopped (preferably Thai basil)

Put the oil in a large stockpot, then add the onion, parsnips, garlic, and ginger and sauté over medium heat until the onions start to look translucent, 5 to 7 minutes. Add in the curry and coriander and cook, stirring constantly, for another minute. Add the sweet potatoes and cook over medium heat for several minutes longer, stirring occasionally. Stir in the peppers, tomatoes, and broth. Bring to a boil, then simmer for at least 30 minutes or until the vegetables have softened.

Remove the soup from the heat, add in the coconut milk, and puree the soup with an immersion blender. You can also blend the soup in small batches in a high-speed blender once it has slightly cooled. Season with salt and pepper and top with basil. Serve hot.

BUTTERNUT SQUASH, FENNEL, AND CARROT SOUP
MAKES 4 TO 5 SERVINGS

The vegetables in this soup provide an abundance of carotenoids. The benefit of carotenoids is that we convert carotene (a plant pigment) into vitamin A to support growth, eye health, and all immune system functions.

- 1 tablespoon olive, coconut, or avocado oil
- 1 yellow onion, roughly chopped
- 3 celery stalks, roughly diced
- 1 fennel bulb, roughly chopped (save fennel fronds)
- 2 teaspoons fresh ginger, grated
- 1 medium butternut squash, peeled and chopped
- 10 to 12 medium carrots, peeled and roughly diced
- 3 to 4 cups vegetable broth
- 1 teaspoon salt
- Bouquet garni of fresh thyme, parsley, and reserved fennel fronds
- ⅓ cup full-fat unsweetened canned coconut milk

Put the oil, onion, celery, and fennel in a large stockpot and sauté for several minutes. Add the ginger and cook for another minute, stirring to incorporate. Stir in the butternut squash, carrots, 3 cups of the broth, and salt. Bring to a boil, then simmer for 40 minutes.

Remove from the heat, add the coconut milk, and puree the soup with an immersion blender. You can also blend the soup in small batches in a high-speed blender once it has slightly cooled. Depending on the thickness of the soup, you may need to add the last cup of broth. Season with salt and pepper to taste and serve hot.

NOTE: After Reset, to increase the soup's nutritional value, think about adding ½ cup dried red lentils and another cup of broth before simmering the soup; lentils are a rich plant-based source of protein.

HEARTY VEGETABLE SOUP
MAKES 8 TO 10 SERVINGS (SEE NOTES)

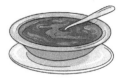

When all is said and done, there is nothing like a hearty soup. The vegetables are tender and the broth is thick and flavorful. The best part of this soup is that you can build on it down the road (after Reset) with lentils and white beans. Add-ins like quinoa or whole-grain buckwheat are highly encouraged. Play around and substitute other vegetables. There is no right or wrong with soup! Soup made at home is far superior to what comes out of a can.

- 2 tablespoons olive, coconut, or avocado oil
- 2 large leeks, trimmed, cleaned, and roughly chopped (tender parts only, discard the tougher outer green part)
- 4 celery stalks, sliced
- 4 large carrots, peeled and sliced
- 4 parsnips, peeled and sliced
- 1 celery root, peeled and chopped
- 1 butternut squash, peeled and chopped
- 4 potatoes of choice, peeled and chopped
- 1 (15-ounce) can diced tomatoes or 2 tomatoes, chopped
- 4 to 5 cups vegetable broth
- 2 tablespoons dried herb blend (vegetable blends, herb and garlic, chimichurri blend, or make your own)
- Bouquet garni of fresh rosemary, thyme, parsley, oregano, or whatever you have
- 1 tablespoon pesto (optional, see notes)

In a large stockpot or Dutch oven, sauté the oil and leeks over medium-high heat, stirring often, for 5 minutes. Stir in the celery, carrots, and parsnips and continue to cook for another 5 minutes. Add the celery root, butternut squash, and potatoes and continue to cook for another 10 minutes, stirring occasionally. Add the tomatoes, 4 cups of the broth, dried herbs, and bouquet garni. At this point, everything should be stirred together, and the broth should be slightly covering the vegetables. If you feel as though you need more, add the remaining 1 cup broth. Cover and simmer for 45 minutes.

Remove from the heat and let sit for at least 30 minutes. Remove the bouquet garni and stir in the pesto (if using). Season with salt and pepper to taste and serve hot.

NOTES: Freezing soup is convenient and time-saving, but please make sure to cool the soup down properly before it goes into the freezer—use an ice bath to quicken the process. Store the cooled soup in a freezer bag and lay it flat if space is an issue, or consider Souper Cubes (see Resources) for convenient freezer-friendly containers. The safest and best way to thaw soup is to place the container in a warm water bath until fully thawed. Place the thawed soup in a pot and reheat on the stovetop over low heat for best results.

Check out the Condiments, Sauces, Dips, and Spreads sections for a pesto recipe to add a pop of flavor to this soup.

SNACKS AND DESSERTS

DATES AND TAHINI
SERVES 1

*A decadent yet healthy way to snack: sweet
and savory, minimal ingredients, and an
array of benefits to curb any sweet tooth.
This treat won't spike your blood sugar
and leave you crashing afterward. Medjool*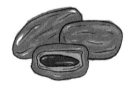
*dates are the best to use for snacking. They are incredibly soft and
wonderful to use in recipes as an alternative to processed sugar.*

- 3 Medjool dates, pitted (see note)
- 1 tablespoon tahini
- Pinch of pink sea salt (optional)
- Swirl of honey (optional)

Cut open the dates and spread the tahini inside. Sprinkle the salt and
drizzle the honey (if using) over the top and enjoy. You can also simply
dip dates in tahini for a quick version.

NOTE: After Reset, continue enjoying this satisfying treat and try
additional add-ins such as nut butter, dark chocolate, or shredded
coconut.

Dried Fruit

Dried fruit is a great source of antioxidants, especially polyphenols, which are associated with better digestive health, improved blood flow, and a decrease in oxidative stress. Polyphenol-rich foods combat inflammation and elevated histamine-related responses. In addition, when we keep our food intake rich in plant phenols, we lower our risk of heart disease, degenerative brain disease, diabetes, and cancer.

Having dried fruit in Reset is a great way to shift away from sugary processed snacks that contribute to excess inflammation in our blood. The antioxidants abundant in this type of snack can help control and reduce blood sugar levels. Many dried fruits are naturally rich in minerals, proteins, fiber, and vitamins and are tasty and satisfying. All in moderation, and don't forget to read your labels, as it is important to avoid added sugars in packaged dried fruits.

My favorite dried fruit is dates because they are a serious candidate for the healthiest dried fruit. They are also a low-glycemic pick, packed with iron, fiber, potassium, and impressive antioxidants. Other low-glycemic dried fruit options are apples, apricots, and plums.

NOTE: If dried fruit makes you gassy, consider smaller quantities. The transformation from fresh fruit to dried concentrates the natural sugars, which can cause bloating if consumed in large quantities. If you are especially gassy, you may be more sensitive and should avoid that particular fruit.

BAKED SEAWEED SNACKS
MAKES ABOUT 6 SERVINGS

Seaweed and its nutritional value are underrated. These tasty sheets pack a higher amount of vitamins and minerals than most vegetables, with impressive amounts of vitamins A and C, calcium, iodine, potassium, selenium, iron, and magnesium.

Making your own seaweed snacks comes with more benefits than just saving money: you can eliminate the inflammatory oils and preservatives often found in commercial brands. Baked at home, quick and easy, low in calories, and topping the charts in nutrients—it's worth giving these addictive treats a try.

- 10 unroasted nori (dried seaweed) sheets
- Olive, coconut, or avocado oil

Preheat the oven to 325°F. Line a baking sheet with parchment paper. Cut the nori lengthwise into 2-inch strips (most nori sheets come with precut lines you can follow) and arrange them smooth side down on the parchment paper. Lightly coat the nori with oil (pump sprays work well) and season with salt. Bake for 12 to 15 minutes until dry and crispy.

Store in an airtight container at room temperature for up to a week or freeze, but don't refrigerate, as this will make them soggy.

NOTE: There are many flavor variations you can try. Brush on tahini with a basting brush, garnish with sesame seeds, or top with dried herbs like za'atar. You may need to add some of the dried spices halfway through cooking, otherwise they may burn.

PUMPKIN BUCKWHEAT CEREAL MUFFINS
MAKES 12 MUFFINS

Cream of Buckwheat cereal is similar to Cream of Wheat and is an excellent alternative for those that are sensitive to oatmeal. You can also use creamy buckwheat cereal (from Bob's Red Mill—the grains are a little thicker), but you may need a little more liquid if the batter gets too thick. Buckwheat is a highly nutritious, easily digested superfood. It is a good source of protein and fiber and contains 8 of the 9 essential amino acids. In addition, minerals such as manganese, magnesium, copper, and zinc help support positive immune system responses.

- 6 tablespoons ground flaxseed
- ⅓ cup water
- ⅔ cup oat or other nondairy milk
- 2 teaspoons vanilla extract
- 3 tablespoons maple syrup
- 1 (15-ounce) can pumpkin puree
- 3 Medjool dates, pitted and chopped into small pieces
- 2 cups Cream of Buckwheat cereal
- 1 teaspoon baking soda
- 1 teaspoon salt
- 1 tablespoon Pumpkin Pie Spice

Preheat the oven to 350°F. Line a muffin pan with baking cups.

In a large bowl, create the flax egg by combining the flaxseed and water and letting it sit for 5 minutes. Then, stir in the oat milk, vanilla, maple syrup, pumpkin puree, and dates. Add the Cream of Buckwheat cereal, baking soda, salt, and Pumpkin Pie Spice and mix well. The consistency should be like cake batter, thick but manageable. You should be able to scoop out portions into your muffin pan easily, filling each cup to the top. Bake for 30 minutes until golden brown. Enjoy straight from the oven!

Store extra muffins in the refrigerator for best results. These muffins can also be frozen.

NOTES: After Reset, consider adding in ¼ cup of any of these optional ingredients: shredded coconut, chocolate chips, cocoa nibs, or dried blueberries (I like the tiny ones at Trader Joe's). Dried blueberries are the only one of these add-ins you can try during Reset.

Once while making these muffins, I ran into the dilemma of not having dates. No problem! I subbed in some dried blueberries and goji berries. On another occasion, I had only half a can of pumpkin, so I added a mashed banana to the mix. Something like applesauce would also work. A lack of ingredients shouldn't throw a wrench in your day (see Plan Your Meals).

OVEN-DRIED MULBERRIES
MAKES ABOUT 8 SERVINGS

Mulberries have a naturally sweet flavor with no added sugar and provide high levels of protein and iron. Mulberries are also a rich source of vitamin C, fiber, calcium, polyphenols, and antioxidants. They tend to be a bit chewy, like raisins, but I dry them out more in my oven to make them extra crunchy. Look for them where the store stocks flaxseed, hempseed, and such. They are great to snack on or you can sprinkle them on top of yogurt (after Reset) or applesauce. I have also ground them up to use in place of graham crackers for pie crusts. It's the new granola!

- 8 ounces mulberries

Preheat the oven to 200°F. Line a baking tray with parchment paper and add the mulberries. Roast for 20 minutes. Remove from the oven and let sit for 10 minutes. They will become nice and crunchy.

Store the dried mulberries in the freezer.

QUICK APPLESAUCE
MAKES ABOUT 2 CUPS

Applesauce is a perfect snack: no added sugar and the cooked apples are easy on the digestive tract. Fresh is so much better and takes only 25 minutes to make. Enjoy this on its own, on top of a toasted muf- 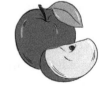 *fin or pancake, or as a layer in a parfait. You can use any apples for sauce, but I recommend using softer apples like Granny Smith, Golden Delicious, or Fuji.*

- 8 apples, peeled and roughly chopped
- ¼ to ½ cup water
- 1 tablespoon ground cinnamon
- Dash of ground nutmeg

In a medium saucepan, combine the apples, ¼ cup of the water, cinnamon, and nutmeg. Bring to a boil, then simmer, letting the juices release for about 15 minutes until the fruit breaks down and the liquids reduce. The apples will become visibly softer and the liquid thicker as the natural sugars release and form a glaze. Add the other ¼ cup water if the liquid dries out completely and your apples are still hard.

Use an immersion blender to blend the applesauce to your desired consistency. You can also blend the applesauce in a high-speed blender or food processor once it has slightly cooled.

FRESH COCONUT SMOOTHIE
MAKES 1 SERVING

Once, at the grocery store, I meant to buy coconut water but accidentally came home with a coconut smoothie. I thought, Oh no, this is going to be a sugar bomb. *I was ecstatic to learn the only 2 ingredients were organic coconut water and fresh coconut meat. It was delicious! So I had to make my own version.*

Coconut, unlike many other fruits that are carb rich, provides us with mostly fat, some protein, and high amounts of manganese, a mineral essential for bone health and the metabolism of carbohydrates, proteins, and cholesterol. Coconut is also rich in copper, iron, and selenium. The fat in coconut is a medium-chain triglyceride (MCT). Our bodies metabolize this type of fat differently than other types because we absorb the fat directly from our small intestine, meaning we can use it rapidly for energy. Coconut oil also inhibits the growth of several strands of bacteria. Therefore, we give it kudos for being antiviral, antifungal, antiprotozoal, and antibacterial. Last but not least, coconut provides our bodies with polyphenol antioxidants, which aid in protecting our cells against damaging oxidative stress. Drink up, it's a great snack or pick-me-up!

- 1 cup coconut water
- ½ cup coconut meat (see notes)

Put both ingredients in a high-speed blender and blend until smooth and creamy.

NOTES: Fresh coconut meat can often be found in the produce aisle and sometimes in the freezer section of the supermarket. Asian markets definitely stock this. Young coconut meat is preferable but not necessary.

A delicious add-in is fresh or frozen papaya. Use ¼ cup coconut and ¼ cup papaya. It's delicious!

FROZEN BANANA CREAM
MAKES 1 SERVING

The benefits of bananas are abundant. They boost digestive health and provide a healthy dose of fiber, protein, and antioxidants. This is an easy and delicious way to use some of your frozen bananas on those nights when you want a frozen treat. With nutrients like magnesium, tryptophan, B6, and potassium, bananas are also linked to improved sleeping habits. Don't overdo it; it's very filling!

- 1 large or 2 small frozen bananas (see note)
- 1 Medjool date, pitted
- ¼ cup oat or other nondairy milk
- 1 to 2 frozen pineapple chunks (optional)

Put all the ingredients in a high-speed blender and blend until smooth. You want a very thick and creamy consistency, like thick soft-serve ice cream. If it's not thick enough, you may want to add a few more pieces of banana. If it's too thick, add a splash more milk.

NOTE: I recommend cutting up the bananas while fresh and freezing them in chunks.

Fruit on the Go

When fruit is prepped, ready, and visible, its chances of being consumed increase dramatically. Grab a couple of glass con- tainers for easy, safe storage, and this smart kitchen strategy will reward you time and time again.

Dice some melon, peel an orange, or cut up an apple. Grab some grapes, berries, and diced mango. How convenient and what a lifesaver in those moments when you are getting ready to run out the door!

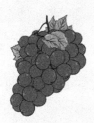 Follow through on meal prep with all your vegetables and fruits—after a trip to the farm, supermarket, or backyard if you are lucky, give them a rinse and store them appropriately. Having ready-to-eat produce will increase the likelihood of your consuming it.

Think of how colorful your refrigerator and countertops will look. Now consider all the healthy fiber, vitamins, minerals, 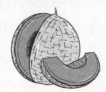 and gut-friendly nutrients you are about to benefit from while becoming so prepared.

CONDIMENTS, SAUCES, DIPS, AND SPREADS

PUMPKIN PIE SPICE
MAKES 1 TABLESPOON

This is a simple way to make your own pumpkin pie spice for sweet and savory dishes.

- 2 teaspoons cinnamon
- ½ teaspoon ground nutmeg
- ½ teaspoon ground ginger

Mix all ingredients in a bowl until combined. Store in an airtight mason jar or container and keep with your everyday herbs.

MIXED HERB PESTO
MAKES ½ CUP

This is a simple and easy way to make a pesto-type sauce for many different uses. This is delicious on any roasted vegetables and especially baked, mashed, or steamed potatoes. You can finish any of the Reset dishes with a drizzle of this pesto to enhance the flavor. I encourage you to make extra and freeze leftovers in ice trays or smaller containers so you always have some on hand. Just a cube or two added to a soup will really make it sing! I've used this pesto in vinaigrettes, as a pizza sauce, and even blended with broth and nondairy cheese to create a creamy pasta sauce.

- 2 cups fresh basil
- Small handful of fresh oregano
- 5 to 6 fresh sage leaves
- 2 sprigs fresh rosemary, stems removed (see notes)
- ¼ cup olive oil

Put all the ingredients in a high-speed blender and blend until you get a thick but smooth consistency. Season with salt and pepper.

NOTES: Char the rosemary before it goes into the blender with a torch or over a stove flame. Just enough to make it crackle and turn brown. This will add a nice smoky flavor and keep the rosemary from overpowering the blend.

I like using a smaller blender cup to make pesto. If there are still remnants of pesto in the blender cup, I take that opportunity to make salad dressing. Don't waste the food in those hard-to-reach areas you can't scrape out.

TARRAGON PESTO
MAKES ½ CUP

Tarragon Pesto can be used in a marinade, soup, or plant-based pasta. It can also give life to a collard wrap or be used as a sandwich spread. The medicinal benefits of tarragon are quite impressive, including its ability to reduce blood sugar and inflammation throughout the body. It is also used medicinally for indigestion, nausea, and toothaches. Its taste is like licorice or fennel but very light and refreshing.

- 1 cup fresh tarragon leaves
- 1 cup fresh parsley

- 1 tablespoon fresh oregano
- 2 tablespoons olive oil
- 2 tablespoons water
- 1 to 2 cloves Roasted Garlic
- 2 tablespoons lemon juice
- ½ teaspoon salt
- ¼ teaspoon pepper

Put all the ingredients in a high-speed blender and blend until you get a thick but smooth consistency.

TAHINI SAUCE
MAKES ¼ CUP

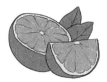

This Asian-inspired sauce is perfect for rice-based dishes or as a stir-fry sauce for vegetables. It can also be used as a dipping sauce for roasted vege-tables or as a creamy salad dressing. Also, this is great served warm or in a cold dish like a noodle salad. Double the recipe if you are using it for a noodle dish or salad feeding four or more.

- 2 tablespoons tahini
- 1 tablespoon lime juice
- 1 tablespoon maple syrup
- 1 tablespoon fresh cilantro, finely chopped
- 1 tablespoon coconut or apple cider vinegar
- 1 teaspoon fresh ginger, grated

Put all the ingredients in a small bowl or mason jar and whisk or shake until well combined.

NOTE: This is a thick sauce, so if you're using it for a hot meal such as rice or buckwheat noodles, pour the sauce on while its hot. For cold meals, you can thin it out with vegetable broth.

SIMPLE SALAD VINAIGRETTE
MAKES 1 CUP

*A little goes a long way with this powerful dressing, as there are many fla-
vors here! I use this so frequently that I make enough to use for the week.
After Reset, consider using this to dress a quick kale or pasta salad.*

- ½ cup water
- ⅓ cup olive oil, or ¼ cup tahini
- ⅓ cup coconut or apple cider vinegar
- 2 tablespoons lime or lemon juice
- 1 teaspoon honey or maple syrup
- 1 teaspoon Dijon mustard
- 1 shallot, chopped
- 1 tablespoon dried herb blend (garlic and herb, chimichurri
  blend, lemon pepper, or tarragon)
- Optional add-ins: fresh herbs, finely chopped (basil, arugula,
  tarragon, cilantro, or parsley)

Put all the ingredients in a blender and blend for 1 minute. Let sit at
room temperature for 10 minutes, then give it a shake to remix prior
to using.

GREEN GODDESS VINAIGRETTE
MAKES 1½ CUPS

*In Reset, this vinaigrette is wonderful added to some roasted potatoes.
Use it as a salad dressing for a simple salad paired with avocado and
cubed sweet potatoes for a complete meal. It is perfect for a cold pasta
salad with buckwheat noodles. Also consider using it in a vegan rice
bowl (see Buddha Bowls) or as a dipping sauce for Collard Green Wraps.*

- ½ cup fresh parsley, chopped
- ⅓ cup fresh basil, chopped
- ¼ cup fresh tarragon, chopped

- ¼ cup olive oil
- ¼ cup water
- 3 tablespoons chives, minced, or ½ shallot, peeled and minced
- 2 tablespoons lemon juice
- ½ teaspoon tomato paste
- 1 teaspoon apple cider vinegar
- 1 teaspoon coconut aminos

Put all the ingredients in a high-speed blender and blend until smooth. Season with salt and pepper. Store in a mason jar in the fridge and shake well before serving.

TAHINI DRESSING OR DIPPING SAUCE
MAKES 1 CUP

Tahini is easy for your body to digest because of its high alkaline mineral content. The phytoestrogens present in tahini are extremely beneficial in managing hormones in women.

To use this as a dressing on any kind of salad, use more water. If you are going to use this as a dipping sauce with a beautiful plate of roasted vegetables (beets, carrots, sweet potatoes), do not use as much water. As a sauce, it works great in Buddha Bowls.

- 1 shallot, roughly chopped
- ¼ cup tahini
- ¼ cup lemon juice
- 3 tablespoons Dijon mustard
- 2 tablespoons nutritional yeast
- 1 tablespoon dried herb blend (garlic and herb or chimichurri), or 3 tablespoons fresh herbs (oregano, tarragon, or charred rosemary)
- 1 Medjool date, pitted, or 2 teaspoons maple syrup
- ¼ to ½ cup water

Put the shallot, tahini, lemon juice, Dijon mustard, nutritional yeast, dried herbs, and date in a high-speed blender and pulse. Add ¼ cup water and blend again. Blend in more water as needed to achieve the proper consistency. Season with salt and pepper. Store in a mason jar in the fridge. The dressing may thicken up when refrigerated, so you may need to remove it from the refrigerator 10 minutes prior to use and give it a good shake.

YUZU PEA PUREE
MAKES 2 CUPS

I am in love with this puree. Yuzu is a citrus fruit juice that is slightly tart yet sweet, fresh, and light. I typically order bottles of this specialty juice online, but I've included a substitution if it's not available.

You can call it a hummus, sauce, or the dash of color your plate needs. Either way, these flavors pair with almost anything: protein, raw or roasted vegetables, rice crackers, or Baked Potato Fries or Chips.

If you want to be extra fancy, you can create a sexy-smooth sauce by pressing the puree through a mesh colander. This is optional and might require extra broth.

- 1 tablespoon olive oil
- 1 shallot, chopped
- 2 cups frozen peas
- 2 cups vegetable broth
- 3 tablespoons yuzu juice, or ½ teaspoon Meyer lemon zest and 3 tablespoons Meyer lemon juice
- 2 ounces dairy-free feta (I like Violife, optional)
- Big handful of baby arugula
- 2 mint leaves
- 20 fresh tarragon leaves

In a medium saucepan, heat the olive oil and sauté the shallot for 2 to 3 minutes, stirring constantly, until it's opaque. Add in the peas and broth. Bring to a low simmer and cook for 2 minutes. Drain, but reserve ⅓ cup of the simmering stock.

Put the cooked peas and shallot, yuzu juice, dairy-free feta, arugula, mint, and tarragon in a food processor. Process on high speed for 1 minute until smooth. If it is too thick, add in some of the reserved vegetable broth a little at a time until you get the desired smooth consistency. Season with salt and pepper to taste. Store in the fridge.

QUICK PICKLED RADISH
MAKES 2 CUPS

Pickling the superfood radish seems a logical thing to do, as in addition to providing a satisfying crunch, pickled radishes detox the body and blood and improve liver and digestive functions. If any types of vinegar give you discomfort, avoid using them in Reset. Coconut vinegar and apple cider vinegar are the mildest versions, so that's what I recommend here. This is a tasty condiment for sushi rolls, veggie burgers, salads, Buddha Bowls, and so much more!

- 8 to 10 radishes, thinly sliced (use a mandolin)
- ¼ red onion, thinly sliced (optional)
- ¾ cup water
- ½ cup coconut or apple cider vinegar
- 2 teaspoons maple syrup
- 1 teaspoon salt
- Pinch of red pepper flakes (optional)
- Optional add-ins: ½ teaspoon mustard seeds, fennel seeds, or peppercorns

Put the radishes and onions (if using) in a mason jar. In a small saucepan, combine the water, coconut vinegar, maple syrup, salt, red pepper flakes (if using), and any optional seasonings. Bring to a boil, then pour the mixture over the radishes and onions. Stir and let sit for 30 minutes. Serve immediately or refrigerate for up to 3 weeks.

NOTE: You may notice that the pickled radishes put off a strong smell after pickling. This is because they are a source of sulfur, so this is to be expected. I recommend storing them in an air-tight mason jar for best results.

BEET SALSA
MAKES 2 TO 3 CUPS

Beets support digestive and brain health with many impressive nutrients. They are also optimal for blood flow and fighting inflammation. There are many different types of beets to choose from such as golden, Chioggia, and striped.

This savory beet salsa is a versatile condiment that complements so many different dishes, such as quinoa and roasted vegetables. One of my favorite pairings for beet salsa is Baked Potato Fries or Chips—I know it sounds a little strange, but you have to try it! I put these two foods together one day out of desperation, and it was a perfect snack that left me full and satisfied. In addition, the digestive benefits are spot-on for a snack.

- 4 medium beets
- 2 shallots or ¼ red onion, diced
- 6 kalamata olives, sliced
- 2 tablespoons lime juice
- 1 tablespoon apple cider vinegar, or 2 tablespoons apple juice
- 1 tablespoon olive oil

You can steam or roast your beets. To steam, fill the bottom of a steamer with about 3 inches of water and bring to a boil. Add the beets to the steamer tray; if you're using larger beets, cut them in half first. Cover and steam for about 15 minutes until tender. Cool, peel, and dice.

To roast, preheat the oven to 400°F. Line a baking sheet with parchment paper. Cut the beets in half (or quarters if they're on the larger side) and lightly coat with oil (pump sprays work well too). Roast for 20 to 25 minutes or until the skins are soft and the beets are tender. Cool, peel, and dice.

To make the salsa, combine the diced beets, shallots, olives, lime juice, apple cider vinegar, and olive oil in a large bowl. Stir to incorporate all the ingredients and season with salt and pepper to taste.

NOTE: After Reset, consider adding in diced apple, golden raisins, jalapeño pepper, and cilantro to serve up the most creative zesty salsa/salad.

CHEF LISA DENIEAR'S CILANTRO-LIME SAUCE
MAKES ABOUT 1 CUP

Chef Lisa, a very dear friend of mine, was kind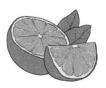
enough to share this delicious recipe with the
world. Thanks, Chef! This recipe is versatile and
can be used as a condiment, marinade, or dress-
ing. It can also be made ahead and frozen for up
to 2 months. I highly encourage using this as a condiment for Collard
Green Wraps or on a baked sweet potato with avocado slices.

- 4 to 5 scallions, green part only, roughly chopped
- 1 bunch fresh cilantro
- Zest of ½ lime (about 1 teaspoon)
- Juice of 2 limes (about ¼ cup)
- 3 tablespoons olive oil
- 2 teaspoons water
- ½ teaspoon salt
- ½ teaspoon ground cumin
- 4 to 7 slices pickled jalapeño (optional)

Put all the ingredients in a high-speed blender and blend until well combined and smooth. Store in a glass container and refrigerate for up to 2 weeks or freeze for up to 2 months.

NO-FAT SALAD DRESSING IN A SNAP
MAKES 1½ CUPS

This dressing is the wonderful invention of two clients who looked all over for a simple dressing with no added fat and could only find a bland soy-based version. We improved it and made it healthier without soy and enhanced the flavors with fresh herbs. If you feel discomfort from the vinegar, save this till after the Reset phase. Into Maintenance and beyond, this should be a staple for so many reasons. It's void of preservatives, artificial flavors, and added sugar alcohols. Recently, I added

some good-quality olive oil and served this over potato salad and on a
cold chickpea and pasta salad. Thanks again, Karen and Laura!

- ⅓ cup water
- ¼ cup coconut or apple cider vinegar
- ¼ cup coconut aminos
- 1 shallot
- Generous handful of herbs of your choice (cilantro, arugula, parsley, dill)
- 2 tablespoons maple syrup
- 2 tablespoons Dijon mustard

Put all the ingredients in a high-speed blender and blend until well combined and smooth. Store in a mason jar in the fridge. You will have to shake it up prior to using it.

WHIPPED TAHINI SAUCE
MAKES ½ CUP

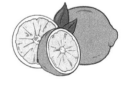

This is a delectable sauce to serve as a condiment, with a salad, or as a dipping sauce with roasted vegetables. For more delicious variations, consider adding fresh herbs such as dill, cilantro, parsley, or basil. It is heavenly with Baked Green Pea Falafel!

- ½ cup tahini
- ¼ cup lemon juice
- ½ teaspoon salt
- Pinch of ground cumin
- ¼ cup hot water

Put all the ingredients in a high-speed blender and blend until well combined and smooth. You may need to add more water, one tablespoon at a time, until you achieve a smooth, creamy consistency. Store in a glass container in the fridge.

FRESH OR FROZEN FRUIT SAUCE
YIELD VARIES

Our intestinal tracts have an easier time digesting fruit when it is broken down, such as through cooking. So this fruit sauce was born! Cook down some fresh or frozen berries, pears, or peaches for a quick, comforting, and nutrient-dense sauce you can add to your buckwheat pancakes. Or make a cooked-fruit parfait with crunchy mulberries on top.

- 2 cups fresh or frozen fruit of choice
- ¼ cup water
- ½ teaspoon ground cinnamon (optional)

In a saucepan, combine all the ingredients and bring to a low simmer. The fruit will break down as the liquids cook out, then reduce. Simmer the fruit for about 10 minutes. At the end of the cooking time, the fruit sauce will get thicker. Remove from the heat.

For a smooth sauce, use an immersion blender to blend the fruits. For a chunkier sauce, take out about half the fruit and blend the rest. You can also blend the sauce in a high-speed blender once it has slightly cooled.

Eat right away while warm. Store extra sauce in a mason jar in the refrigerator or freezer.

ROASTED GARLIC
YIELD VARIES

Roasting garlic is easy and adds a pop of rich flavor to any savory condiment, soup, or meal. I like to roast a whole bulb or two of garlic so I have plenty when I want to use it.

- 1 or more whole garlic bulbs
- 1 to 2 tablespoons olive oil

Preheat the oven to 375°F. Cut off the end of the bulb opposite the root, exposing the tops of the cloves. Keep the skin on. Coat the whole bulb with 1 to 2 tablespoons of oil and wrap it in foil or parchment paper. Put it on a baking sheet or small pan and roast for 30 to 35 minutes. The garlic smell will fill your home and the garlic will be golden brown and very soft.

When slightly cooled, squeeze out the cloves—they should come right out and be butter-like. You can easily turn the roasted cloves into a paste with a fork (see Verde Pico de Gallo and Nondairy Cheesy Parsnip Sauce). Freeze what you don't use right away.

CHAPTER 14

Maintenance Recipes

BREAKFAST

PINEAPPLE COCONUT SMOOTHIE
MAKES 1 SERVING

This tropical drink offers an array of health benefits, antioxidants, and nutrients. Tropical fruits are beneficial for our digestive tract and help control blood pressure.

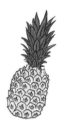

- ½ fresh or frozen banana
- 4 to 5 pieces frozen pineapple
- ¼ cup unsweetened coconut, shredded
- ½ cup coconut water
- ½ cup water or nondairy milk
- Splash of lime juice
- 2 tablespoons ground hempseed, ground flaxseed, or protein powder (optional)
- Toasted coconut (optional)

Put the banana, pineapple, shredded coconut, coconut water, water, lime juice, and hempseed in a high-speed blender and blend until well combined and smooth. The consistency is up to you, but if you're using a fresh banana, you may want to add less water. Pour into a glass and top with toasted coconut (if using). Enjoy immediately.

SALTED CHOCOLATE DATE SMOOTHIE WITH A TWIST
MAKES 1 SERVING

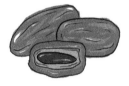

This can be a quick pick-me-up smoothie or the base of a yummy power bowl. When made into a bowl, you can add sliced banana, berries, or shredded coconut on top.

- ½ cup frozen riced cauliflower
- 3 soft Medjool dates, pitted
- 1 tablespoon tahini
- 2 teaspoons unsweetened cacao powder or cocoa
- 2 teaspoons pomegranate powder, or acai, goji, or other super-food powder
- 1 scoop plant-based protein powder
- 1 teaspoon vanilla extract
- ½ cup water or coconut water
- Pinch of salt

Put all the ingredients in a high-speed blender and blend until smooth and creamy. Pour into a glass and enjoy immediately.

SALTED CARAMEL PUMPKIN SMOOTHIE
MAKES 1 SERVING

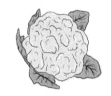

If immune health is a top priority, the benefits of the pumpkin in this smoothie should make this a staple in your routine. One-half cup of canned pumpkin offers about 3.5 grams of healthful fiber in addition to plenty of beta-carotene, vitamins C and E, iron, and folate. Riced cauliflower is a secret cruciferous vegetable addition that is naturally high in fiber and B vitamins. Cauliflower is considered a superfood because it's nutrient rich and has a high antioxidant content.

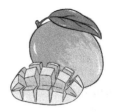

*When our immune system is properly sup-
ported, our cells are better equipped to ward off
germs and speed up healing when invaders are
present. Make this smoothie as a drink, or use
less ice to create a thicker base for a bowl topped
with fresh fruit and granola. I do suggest trying
this with a tablespoon of almond butter or subbing half the amount of
nondairy milk for canned coconut milk. Both are delicious additions
that make a creamier smoothie.*

- ½ cup canned pumpkin (see notes)
- 2 Medjool dates, pitted
- 3 to 4 pieces frozen mango (see notes)
- ½ cup frozen riced cauliflower
- 2 ice cubes
- ¾ cup oat or other nondairy milk
- ½ teaspoon Pumpkin Pie Spice
- ½ teaspoon vanilla extract
- Pinch of sea salt
- 2 tablespoons ground hempseed or ground flaxseed, or
  1 serving protein powder (optional, see notes)

Put all the ingredients in a high-speed blender and blend until well
combined and smooth. Enjoy immediately.

NOTES: If it's available, you can also use freshly cooked pumpkin,
but make sure it is cooled and note that you may need a little more
milk, as fresh pumpkin can be starchier.

In place of mango, you can substitute any frozen fruit, but I've
found mango works best, as it does not take away from the pumpkin
flavor. To mix it up, cherries are yummy, and bananas are delicious but
will be the dominant flavor.

Please see the recommended brands of protein powders under
Pantry Nice-to-Haves, as there are many gastrointestinal side effects
associated with brands containing whey (dairy), sugar alcohols, additives, fillers, and preservatives.

CARROT-COCONUT PANCAKES
MAKES ABOUT 20 PANCAKES (SEE NOTE)

This is the perfect combination of nutrients like omega-3s, beta-carotene, and fiber and is a tasty and filling breakfast or breakfast-for-dinner treat.

- 5 tablespoons ground flaxseed
- 2 cups water, divided
- 2 cups oat or other nondairy milk
- 1 cup unsweetened applesauce
- 2 tablespoons maple syrup
- 2 cups carrots, shredded (4 to 5 carrots)
- 1½ cups organic rice flour
- 1 cup buckwheat flour
- ¼ cup coconut flour
- ¼ cup coconut, grated
- 1 tablespoon Pumpkin Pie Spice
- 1 tablespoon baking powder
- ½ teaspoon salt
- Coconut, avocado, or olive oil
- Fresh fruit, maple syrup, or maple cream (optional)

In a large bowl, create the flax egg by combining ½ cup of the water with the ground flaxseed and letting it sit for 5 minutes. Add the remaining 1½ cups water, oat milk, applesauce, maple syrup, and carrots and stir to incorporate.

In a smaller bowl, combine the rice flour, buckwheat flour, coconut flour, grated coconut, Pumpkin Pie Spice, baking powder, and salt and stir to combine. Add the dry ingredients to the wet and stir until well mixed.

Lightly coat a frying pan or griddle with oil (pump sprays work well too). Use about ¼ cup batter for each pancake. Cook over medium-high heat, flip after 3 to 4 minutes, then cook for another 2 to 3 minutes until the pancakes are set. Reapply oil as needed and work through all the batter to make extras to freeze. Now you are super prepared! Serve hot with the toppings of your choice.

NOTE: This is a large recipe, so if you don't eat all the pancakes, the extras can be frozen and reheated in a snap on the stovetop or in the microwave.

SWEET POTATO MUFFINS
MAKES 12 MUFFINS

These muffins are super moist, nutrient dense, and delicious. The lack of added sugars helps balance blood sugar and regulate insulin. Hemp and flaxseed act as binders and offer complete protein, minerals, and omegas. In addition, buckwheat flour is a superfood and a great source of protein, fiber, and minerals. I've used cooked or canned BPA-free sweet potatoes on different occasions. The canned potato version saves time and produces a lighter muffin. The fresh potato version is a little denser but equally delicious.

- ¼ cup ground flaxseed
- ¼ cup hemp hearts
- ⅓ cup water
- ⅓ cup coconut oil, melted
- ⅓ cup maple syrup
- 1 teaspoon vanilla extract
- 1½ cups cooked and roughly mashed sweet potato, or 1 (15-ounce) can sweet potatoes
- 1 cup oat or other nondairy milk
- 1 cup buckwheat flour
- ¾ cup almond meal
- ¼ cup coconut flour
- 1 teaspoon ground ginger
- 1 teaspoon Pumpkin Pie Spice
- 1 teaspoon baking soda
- 1 teaspoon baking powder
- 6 carrots, shredded
- 1 apple, shredded
- ¼ cup unsweetened coconut, shredded
- ¼ cup golden raisins

Preheat the oven to 350°F.

In a large bowl, create the flax egg by combining the flaxseed, hemp hearts, and water and letting it sit for 5 minutes.

Add the coconut oil, maple syrup, vanilla, sweet potato, and oat milk to the bowl. Mix well with a whisk. Add the buckwheat flour, almond meal, coconut flour, ground ginger, Pumpkin Pie Spice, baking soda, and baking powder and stir until well incorporated. Fold the carrots, apple, coconut, and golden raisins into the mixture.

Line a muffin pan with liners and fill each three-quarters full of batter. Bake for 35 to 40 minutes until set and browned. Eat right away or refrigerate for up to a week. Freeze any extras.

BUCKWHEAT BAGELS
MAKES ABOUT 1 DOZEN MINI-BAGELS

It is rewarding to finally come up with a bagel recipe that is chewy, vegan, and gluten-free. This recipe calls for lots of blueberries and pumpkin seeds. The wild blueberries are packed with nutrients and antioxidants that aid in building strong immune systems. Pumpkin seeds contain a considerable amount of vitamins E and B complex, magnesium, zinc, and omega-3s. They are also an excellent source of tryptophan, which is critical for a good night's sleep.

I highly recommend using your hands to knead this mixture well. It is not your typical gluten filled recipe. It may look dry when you are mixing it; it should resemble a thick cookie dough–type of mixture.

- 2 cups buckwheat flour
- ⅓ cup coconut flour
- ¾ cup arrowroot flour
- 1 teaspoon cinnamon or Pumpkin Pie Spice
- 1½ teaspoons kosher salt
- 2 cups warm water (about 110°F)
- 1 tablespoon highly active yeast
- ¼ cup maple syrup
- 2 tablespoons coconut oil, melted

- ½ cup ground flaxseed
- ¼ cup hemp hearts
- 2 cups blueberries (see note)
- ¼ cup toasted pumpkin seeds
- Silicone mini-bagel tray

In a large bowl, combine the buckwheat flour, coconut flour, arrowroot flour, cinnamon, and salt.

In a big glass bowl, combine the warm water, yeast, and maple syrup. Let stand for a minute and then mix to combine. Add the coconut oil, flaxseed, and hemp hearts. Whisk to combine and let the mixture sit for no more than 2 minutes or it will get too gelatinous.

Slowly add the wet ingredients to the dry, mixing as you pour. I recommend using disposable gloves and mixing with your hands. Add the blueberries and pumpkin seeds and knead all the ingredients for about 3 minutes. The mixture will turn dark from the blueberry juice and resemble a very thick dough.

Fill the silicone mini-bagel tray with the dough. If you don't have one of these, you can also line a baking sheet with parchment paper and form the dough into bagels by hand. Take about ¼ cup of the dough and form it into the shape of a bagel. Use your finger to make the hole in the middle.

Let the bagels rise for 40 minutes. If you are lucky enough to have a humid day, that is ideal, or you can use the bread-proofing function on your oven, which is between 75°F and 90°F.

About 20 minutes before the bagels are done rising, preheat the oven to 400°F. Bake the bagels for 35 to 40 minutes. Cool for an additional 10 to 15 minutes.

I highly recommend toasting the bagels before serving if you are not eating them right out of the oven. Store extra bagels in an airtight container and refrigerate up to a week. If freezing extras, I recommend preslicing the bagels for convenience, as this time-saving trick will be helpful when thawing.

NOTE: At times, I have switched up the blueberries for mashed bananas or added both. Either or both are essential because they add flavor as well as moisture.

LUNCH AND DINNER

EGG ROLL NOODLE BOWLS
MAKES 2 SERVINGS

In this dish, rice noodles take the place of your typical wonton wrapper. If you can find forbidden rice noodles, try them out to add a colorful pop to a delicious meal. Either way, there are many different types of rice and vegetable-based noodles for those with celiac or gluten sensitivities.

This healthy meal in one is a delicious way to reap the benefits of plant-based superfoods. There are vitamins, minerals, and nutrients galore, plus changing the vegetable lineup is a creative way to reinvent this bowl again and again.

- 4 ounces purple or brown rice noodles or buckwheat noodles
- ½ cup frozen edamame or lima beans
- 2 tablespoons olive, coconut, or avocado oil
- ½ yellow onion, sliced
- ½ head small green or napa cabbage, shredded
- 1 large carrot, julienned or thinly sliced
- 1 cup mushrooms, diced
- 1 cup broccoli florets, broccolini, or broccoli rabe
- ¼ cup coconut aminos
- 2 tablespoons sweet chili sauce (see note)
- Scallions, chopped
- Sesame seeds
- Spicy Chickpea Tahini Sauce (see Quinoa Vegetable Sushi)

Cook the noodles according to the package directions. Rinse with cool water and set aside. Blanch the edamame in boiling salted water for 3 minutes, then rinse and set aside.

Put the oil, onion, cabbage, and carrot in a large skillet. Sauté over medium heat for several minutes, stirring constantly. Add the mushrooms and broccoli and cook for several more minutes, stirring so they cook evenly. If the mushrooms release a lot of water, sauté until most of the water has evaporated. Add the coconut aminos and chili sauce and incorporate evenly into the vegetables.

If needed, warm up the noodles and edamame in the skillet over low heat. Layer each bowl with the vegetable mixture, noodles, and edamame. Top with the Spicy Chickpea Tahini Sauce and garnish with the scallions and sesame seeds. Serve immediately.

NOTE: If you don't have a sweet chili sauce, whip up your own with 2 parts hot sauce to 1 part honey.

MEXICAN RICE BOWLS
MAKES 2 SERVINGS

Remember our Buddha Bowls? Take it up a notch and get creative with a Mexican-inspired bowl where rice or quinoa are balanced with refried beans, sautéed greens, peppers, and toppings such as fresh avocado. If you have leftover filling, consider freezing it to turn Green Lentil Lasagna into a Mexican inspired lasagna. It would also be delicious in a quesadilla!

- 1 tablespoon olive, coconut, or avocado oil
- ¼ red onion, diced
- 1 red or green bell pepper, diced or cut into long strips
- 1 teaspoon Taco Seasoning
- ¼ cup water
- 1 cup refried beans
- 2 cups baby greens (spinach, kale, Swiss chard, or a combination)
- ½ cup cilantro, chopped
- ½ cup mild or spicy salsa

- ⅔ cup cooked wild or brown rice or quinoa
- Optional toppings: salsa, jalapeños, nondairy shredded cheese, diced avocado, Baked Tortilla Strips (see sidebar)

Put the oil, onions, and bell peppers in a large skillet or pan and cook over medium heat for 5 minutes, stirring occasionally. Add in the Taco Seasoning and water and cook, stirring to incorporate, for 2 to 3 minutes. Add the refried beans and break them up in the mixture. Then add the baby greens, cilantro, and salsa and mix well. Continue to cook for 10 more minutes until all greens are wilted and the mixture is heated though. Remove from the heat.

To serve, split the rice between the bowls and top with the bean mixture and optional toppings.

Baked Tortilla Strips
MAKES 2 TO 3 SERVINGS

Tortillas cut up into long strips, seasoned, and baked in the oven are a delicious and crunchy garnish. When you make your own, you control the use of the inflammatory oils and GMO ingredients that are so often found in premade versions. You may also want to experiment with grain-free or non-GMO corn tortillas. Store leftovers in an airtight container.

- 2 tortillas
- Olive, coconut, or avocado oil pump spray
- Dried herbs (optional)

Preheat the oven to 350°F. Line a baking pan with parchment paper.

Cut each tortilla into strips about 3 inches in length and place them on the parchment paper. Using the pump spray, lightly coat the strips with oil, then season them with salt, pepper, and dried herbs (if using). Bake for 15 to 20 minutes until the strips are lightly browned. Let cool before using.

LENTILS, VEGGIES, AND RICE WITH TAHINI SAUCE
MAKES 6 TO 8 SERVINGS

This is the perfect meal for when you start introducing beans back into your routine, because these tiny legumes are easy on the digestive tract. This meal also scores high in nutritional value. Lentils contain power-house plant-based nutrients such as protein and fiber and are a great source of B vitamins, iron, magnesium, folate, potassium, and zinc. Rice and lentils is a typical vegan, gluten-free meal, but this takes it to a higher level with riced vegetables added in. Buying frozen riced vegetables is a huge time-saver, so I always encourage stocking up to help yourself out in a pinch.

- 3 tablespoons olive, coconut, or avocado oil, divided
- 2 (12-ounce) bags frozen, thawed, or 6 cups fresh vegetables, riced (broccoli, cauliflower, or sweet potato)
- 1 yellow or red onion, diced
- 1 teaspoon ground cumin
- 1 cup brown lentils
- 1 teaspoon salt
- 2 bay leaves
- 3 cups vegetable broth
- 1 cup wild or brown rice (also look for red, pink, or green organic rice blends)
- Fresh parsley, chopped
- Lemon wedges

TAHINI SAUCE:

- ¼ cup water
- 3 tablespoons tahini
- 2 tablespoons nutritional yeast
- 1 tablespoon lemon juice

Preheat the oven to 350°F. Line a baking sheet with parchment paper and coat with about 2 tablespoons of the oil (pump sprays work well too). Add the riced vegetables.

I usually cook them for 35 to 40 minutes, moving the vegetables around every 15 to 20 minutes, to evaporate the excess water and get a finished product that is golden brown and slightly crunchy. If using fresh riced vegetables, you can sauté them in a pan instead (sautéing frozen riced vegetables tends to make them very mushy and will change the outcome of your dish). Set aside when done.

While the riced vegetables are cooking, put the remaining 1 tablespoon oil and the onion in a large pot and sauté over medium heat for 2 to 3 minutes. Then add the cumin and continue to sauté for another 2 to 3 minutes, stirring constantly so that the cumin does not stick or burn. Add the lentils, salt, bay leaves, and vegetable broth. Bring to a boil, cover, and let simmer for 10 minutes. Add the rice, stir, cover, and simmer for an additional 12 to 15 minutes or until the rice is cooked. Remove from the heat and let sit for an additional 5 minutes. Fold in the cooked riced vegetables.

To make the sauce, put all the sauce ingredients in a high-speed blender or blender cup and blend until well combined and creamy.

Top the vegetable mixture with the Tahini Sauce, parsley, and a squeeze of fresh lemon juice. Season with salt and pepper to taste. Leftovers can be frozen.

QUESADILLAS
MAKES 2 SERVINGS

The beauty of a quesadilla is that you can add almost anything to it and create a meal in minutes. Though this recipe is for 2 servings, this is just a guide. Customize your quesadillas with healthy fillings depending on what leftover vegetables you have.

- 2 cups cooked vegetables of choice, chopped into bite-size pieces
- ¾ cup (about ⅓ can) refried beans
- ¾ cup salsa
- ¼ to ½ cup nondairy cheese (optional)
- Olive, coconut, or avocado oil pump spray
- 4 tortillas

- Optional toppings: salsa, lime wedges, guacamole (or diced avocado)

Put the vegetables, refried beans, salsa, and cheese (if using) in a large mixing bowl and stir well to combine.

Spray a frying pan with oil and heat over medium heat. Add a tortilla and let it heat up for about a minute. Spread about one-quarter of the vegetable mixture evenly on one side of the tortilla and fold it over. Let the tortilla brown and the cheese melt, then flip and brown the other side. Repeat with the rest of the tortillas. Serve hot with the toppings of your choice. Extra quesadillas can be refrigerated; just reheat them on the stovetop to crisp them up.

Quesadilla Combinations

- Sautéed spinach, mushrooms, and onions with nondairy feta
- Sautéed mushrooms, grilled eggplant, and peppers with thinly sliced red onion
- Grilled squash, fresh arugula, and sweet potato
- Roasted broccoli, black beans, and corn
- Caramelized onion and bell peppers
- Sautéed cabbage and mushrooms with jalapeño

WHAT A VEGGIE BURGER!
MAKES 12 BURGERS

This recipe is from my first book, but it has been changed up a bit to include a soy-free and gluten-free glaze for the burger. This is a great recipe to make extras to freeze. Being able to pop this precooked burger out of the freezer for a quick meal is a huge time-saver. My recipe is also void of all the additives, fillers, and preservatives most store-bought veggie burgers contain. My favorite way to eat this burger is hot on top of a salad—it is the perfect meal! No need for a bun either. This is delicious all by itself paired with a slice of avocado and some Whipped Tahini Sauce or Chef Lisa DeNiear's Cilantro-Lime Sauce. I say go for some Quick Pickled Radish while you are at it. You can also serve it with Shaved Brussels Sprout Salad with Lemon-Shallot Vinaigrette or Fennel Coleslaw with Grapefruit Dressing. See the Veggie Burger Wraps recipe for a way to use this burger in a creative and delicious wrap.

GLAZE:

- 3 tablespoons molasses
- 3 tablespoons coconut aminos
- 2 tablespoons coconut aminos hoisin sauce (see notes)
- 2 tablespoons honey

BURGERS:

- 1 cup carrots, grated (see notes)
- 1 large zucchini, shredded
- 2 (15-ounce) cans black beans, well rinsed, or 3½ cups home-cooked
- 2 cups cooked brown rice
- 1 cup cooked quinoa
- 1 cup cooked beets, chopped
- ½ cup oats
- ½ cup Cream of Buckwheat cereal or ½ cup oats
- ½ red onion, chopped
- 1 tablespoon pickled jalapeño pepper, finely chopped (optional)
- 1 tablespoon red chili powder
- 1 teaspoon salt
- 1 teaspoon black pepper
- 1 teaspoon ground cumin
- 2 tablespoons olive, avocado, or coconut oil

To make the glaze, whisk together all the glaze ingredients in a small bowl.

To make the burgers, in a large bowl, combine all the burger ingredients except the oil. Add half the glaze and mix well with your hands. Take about half the mixture and pulse for a couple of seconds in a food processor (or blender). Add it back to the bowl and mix until well combined. Let the mixture sit for twenty minutes.

Preheat the oven to 350°F.

Line a roasting pan with parchment paper and coat with the oil (pump sprays work well too). Using about ⅓ cup of the mixture each, form burger patties with your hands, pushing the ingredients together tightly. They should be about the size of your palm.

With a basting brush or spoon, coat the top of each burger with the remaining glaze. Put the burgers in the oven and cook for 25 minutes. Then flip the burgers and cook for an additional 20 minutes. If you like a crunchier patty, cook for an additional 10 minutes. Once cooled, you can freeze extras to save for another time.

NOTES: Not sure where to find coconut aminos hoisin sauce? Sourcing this earthy soy-free alternative to hoisin sauce is not difficult. Look in the Asian section of your supermarket. Coconut Secret brand carries many soy-free alternatives.

You can get creative with the veggies for this recipe. For example, I did not have fresh carrots or zucchini recently and substituted a bag of cooked frozen peas and carrots. It worked out beautifully.

VEGGIE BURGER WRAPS
MAKES 2 SERVINGS

This combination is the perfect superfood wrap. Don't feel that you need to follow the recipe exactly; a veggie wrap offers a wonderful way to use up any leftover vegetables and reap their benefits. Also, use ideas from the What a Veggie Burger! recipe to create unique wrap combinations.

- 2 brown rice tortillas or other tortillas of choice (see notes)
- 1 cup fresh salad greens

- 2 tablespoons fresh herbs of choice (basil, cilantro, dill, or tarragon)
- ¼ cup Chef Lisa DeNiear's Cilantro-Lime Sauce (optional)
- 1 What a Veggie Burger! patty
- ½ avocado, smashed
- 6 small pieces sweet potato, cubed, roasted or boiled

In a frying pan over medium-high heat, warm up a tortilla. Move it around and flip it for up to 20 seconds. The tortilla will heat up right away, making it warm and pliable. Quickly add your ingredients to the bottom middle part of the tortilla. Fold over the sides gently and then roll it like a burrito. Repeat with the second tortilla.

NOTES: For the brown rice tortillas, look in the gluten-free freezer section.

Save any leftover wraps for lunch the next day! I recommend cutting the wrap in half and wrapping it in parchment paper to keep it from drying out.

VEGETARIAN LENTIL MEATBALLS
MAKES 20 TO 24 MEATBALLS

Lentils are the base of these meatballs and provide an excellent amount of six important minerals, two B vitamins, protein, and fiber with virtually no fat. I used brown lentils in this recipe but have also substituted red and black lentils with great results. If you are just beginning Maintenance, you can substitute eggplant for the lentils if you don't feel you are ready to handle beans yet. Quinoa is a grain-like seed with an impressive complete protein content; it is also a good source of dietary fiber and is high in magnesium and iron. This gluten-free grain has a crunchy, nutty flavor that is easy to digest.

The meatballs can be eaten on their own with a quick sauce (see recipe in the sidebar or try them with Whipped Tahini Sauce), paired with zucchini noodles, broken up into sauce like a vegan Bolognese, put on top of a salad, added to Buddha Bowls, or used as filling for a wrap with avocado. The possibilities are endless!

- 2 tablespoons olive, coconut, or avocado oil
- 6 tablespoons ground flaxseed
- ½ cup water
- 2 cups cooked lentils or well-rinsed canned lentils (see notes)
- ½ cup fresh spinach, sautéed and chopped (see notes)
- 1 cup zucchini, shredded or grated
- 2 tablespoons tomato paste, or 1 tablespoon Sun-Dried Tomato Spread
- 1 cup cooked quinoa
- ¼ cup fresh herbs, chopped (basil, oregano), or 2 tablespoons dried herb blend (chimichurri blend)
- 1 teaspoon salt
- ½ teaspoon pepper
- Quick Tomato Sauce (optional, see sidebar)

Preheat the oven to 375°F. Line a baking sheet with parchment paper and coat with oil (pump sprays work well too).

In a small bowl, create the flax egg by combining the flaxseed and water and letting it sit for 5 minutes.

In a large bowl, combine the flax egg, lentils, spinach, zucchini, tomato paste, quinoa, herbs, salt, and pepper. Put half the mixture in a food processor and process on medium speed for 2 minutes. Then add it back to the large bowl and recombine. Using your hands, form meatballs about 2 inches in diameter. Place the meatballs on the prepared baking sheet about 2 inches apart.

Put the meatballs in the oven and cook for about 25 minutes. Then flip them and cook for an additional 20 minutes. The meatballs should be browned and have a crunchy outside coating.

NOTES: You can substitute 2 cups of roasted and chopped eggplant for the lentils. Or use 1 cup of each and enjoy the flavors of both!

For the spinach, 8 ounces of fresh spinach will yield ½ cup when cooked. If you are using frozen chopped spinach, 5 ounces will yield about ½ cup after cooking. Squeeze out excess water with a paper towel after it cools.

Quick Tomato Sauce
MAKES ABOUT 2 CUPS

- 2 tablespoons olive oil
- 1 shallot, diced
- 1 (28-ounce) can petite diced tomatoes
- 1 teaspoon tomato paste
- 1 teaspoon capers
- ½ teaspoon dried oregano
- ½ teaspoon dried basil

Put the olive oil and shallots in a small saucepan and cook over medium heat, stirring occasionally, for 2 to 3 minutes. Add in the tomatoes, tomato paste, capers, oregano, and basil. Bring to a simmer and cook for 30 minutes over low heat. Season with salt and pepper to taste.

BUCKWHEAT RAMEN NOODLE STIR-FRY
MAKES 2 SERVINGS

Buckwheat ramen noodles are a delicious, nutritious alternative to ramen noodles, which are typically fried and void of nutrients. Buckwheat (wheat-free and derived from a plant in the rhubarb family) has a rich, nutty flavor and is high in protein and iron. The *noodles are easy to prepare and may end up as a staple in your pantry. The vegetables can be changed up to include any variety that holds up in a stir-fry.*

SAUCE:

- 1 tablespoon tahini
- 1 tablespoon maple syrup or raw honey
- 1 tablespoon coconut aminos

- 1 teaspoon red chili sauce or 1 teaspoon tomato paste and ¼ teaspoon cayenne pepper
- ½ teaspoon fresh ginger, grated

NOODLES:

- 2 tablespoons olive, coconut, or avocado oil
- 1 red bell pepper, thinly sliced
- 1½ cups sugar snap peas, trimmed and halved (see notes)
- ½ onion, diced
- 1½ cups broccoli
- 1 (8-ounce) can water chestnuts, well rinsed and diced
- 2 packs (about 5 ounces) buckwheat ramen noodles (see notes)
- ½ cup vegetable broth
- ½ cup full-fat unsweetened canned coconut milk
- Optional toppings: chopped scallions, chopped cilantro, toasted sesame seeds

To make the sauce, in a small bowl, combine all the sauce ingredients and whisk to incorporate.

In a large wok or cast-iron pan over medium heat, heat the oil and then add the pepper, peas, onion, broccoli, and water chestnuts. Cook, stirring constantly for 4 to 5 minutes. Put the cooked vegetables in a bowl and set aside. Don't clean the wok just yet.

Cook the ramen noodles according to the package directions (I lean more toward al dente so they do not become too mushy), rinse with cold water, and set aside.

In the same wok over medium heat, add the sauce and stir until it gets hot. Then add the vegetable broth and coconut milk and stir to incorporate. Carefully fold in the cooled ramen noodles followed by the vegetables. Mix well and remove from the heat. Garnish with the toppings of your choice and serve immediately.

NOTES: Wondering how to trim a snap pea? It's important because eating a snap pea with the vein intact is unpleasant and hard to chew. The tip or string should be dangling and attached to the concave side of the shell. Use a small paring knife to grab the string and pull along the side. It will come off easily. Once you pull off the first tip, pull the second tip in the opposite direction and discard.

Look for 100 percent buckwheat noodles. King Soba brand is organic and has a 9.8-ounce package that's enough for 4 servings. There are also soup mixes (Lotus Foods, Big Green, and Onetang) with millet and brown rice noodles; just omit the soup seasoning packet and use the noodles.

GREEN LENTIL LASAGNA
MAKES 6 SERVINGS

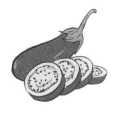

There is a gluten-free brand of lasagna noodles I love—Explore Cuisine—when I'm in the mood for that sort of comfort food. It's a great nutritious noodle, but you can substitute other plant-based noodles.

When making lasagna, there is always room to get creative, especially when adding in roasted vegetables. Just remember to cook down the vegetables first, otherwise your lasagna might become too watery in the oven. Mushrooms can be cooked down and chopped up to create a nice meat substitute in this meal if eggplant is not appealing. Peppers and onions or grilled summer squash with lots of herbs could also take the place of the eggplant. It all comes together in a lasagna. This is also a great recipe to use up your herbs! They are so good for removing pathogens and bacteria from your body.

- Olive, coconut, or avocado oil pump spray
- 1 (25-ounce) jar marinara sauce of your choice
- 1 (8-ounce) box Explore Cuisine Organic Green Lentil Lasagna noodles or other plant-based noodles made from rice, almond flour, or hearts of palm
- 3 cups roasted eggplant, roughly chopped (see notes)
- ½ cup almond ricotta (optional, see notes)
- 2 cups Roasted Cauliflower and Butternut Squash Sauce (see notes)

- 1 teaspoon dried oregano or dried Italian herb blend
- ½ cup crumbled nondairy mozzarella (I like Violife, optional)
- Fresh basil or oregano (optional)

Preheat the oven to 375°F.

Use a pump spray to lightly coat a 10 x 14-inch oven-safe baking dish with oil. Pour in enough marinara sauce to coat the bottom. Cover the sauce with a layer of green lentil noodles. It is okay to break some of them up to make them fit. Layer on the rest of the ingredients as follows, but remember, this is lasagna; it does not have to be perfect! Add 1 to 1½ cups of your roasted vegetables on top of the pasta and spread them out as evenly as possible. Dollop some ricotta (if using) on top of the vegetables. Add 1 to 1½ cups of the sauce on top. Follow the sauce with another layer of noodles and then whatever vegetables you have left. Put any remaining noodles on top.

Top with a combination of the remaining marinara sauce and Roasted Cauliflower and Butternut Squash Sauce, then sprinkle on the dried herbs.

Cover the lasagna with parchment paper and wrap foil tightly across the top. Cook for 40 to 45 minutes. It is done when the noodles are soft. Remove from the oven and add fresh herbs and nondairy mozzarella (if using). Let the lasagna rest for about 10 minutes before serving.

NOTES: To roast the eggplant, first remove the skin. From there, cut

the eggplant in half lengthwise and then across into 1-inch-wide pieces. Salt the pieces and lay them in a colander for 10 to 15 minutes to sweat them. Rinse and dry them off with a paper towel. Lay the eggplant pieces on a large baking pan lined with parchment paper and lightly sprayed with oil. Roast them in the oven at 375°F for 20 to 25 minutes, until nicely browned. Let cool, then chop up into small pieces.

If you are just starting Maintenance, skip the almond ricotta for now.

Make this into a Mexican inspired lasagna by replacing the Roasted Cauliflower and Butternut Squash Sauce with leftover filling from Vegetable Enchiladas or Mexican Rice Bowls.

MEXICAN BAKED POTATOES
MAKES 4 SERVINGS

When thinking about baked potatoes, don't just im-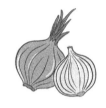
mediately reach for russet. Experiment with all kinds
of potatoes—sweet, yam, white Japanese, even pur-
ple. Did you know that the people of Okinawa, Japan,
attribute living to one hundred years old and beyond to their love of
the purple yam? They consume about a pound of purple potatoes per
day! This gorgeous root vegetable boasts antioxidant levels 150 percent
higher than blueberries.

- 2 medium or large potatoes, any variety
- 1 tablespoon olive, coconut, or avocado oil
- ¼ red onion, diced
- 1 red or green bell pepper, diced
- 1 teaspoon Taco Seasoning
- ¼ cup water
- 1 (15-ounce) can refried beans
- ½ cup fresh cilantro, chopped
- ½ cup mild or spicy salsa
- Optional toppings: salsa, jalapeños, nondairy cheese, diced avocado

Preheat the oven to 425°F. Line a baking sheet with foil or parchment paper.

Scrub the potatoes thoroughly. Prick each several times with a fork to allow steam to release during the cooking process. Lay the potatoes on the prepared baking sheet and put it in the oven. Bake for 50 to 60 minutes, flipping the potatoes every 20 minutes or so and checking for doneness by piercing them with a fork. The potatoes are done when the skins are dry and the insides are completely soft. When the potatoes are finished, remove them from the oven but turn the oven down to 350°F.

While the potatoes bake, combine the oil, onion, and bell pepper in a large pan. Sauté over medium-high heat for several minutes until the onion is translucent, stirring occasionally. Add the Taco

Seasoning and water and stir until most of the water has evaporated and the mixture has thickened. Remove from the heat and put the contents into a large bowl. Add the refried beans, cilantro, and salsa. Stir well to incorporate.

When the potatoes have cooled, cut them in half and use a fork to loosen up the insides. Top the potatoes with the prepared filling, using about ½ cup per potato half. Bake for 25 to 30 minutes until hot. Garnish with toppings of your choice.

CRYSTAL'S CAULIFLOWER PIZZA
MAKES 1 LARGE PIZZA CRUST

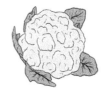

Cauliflower is a wonderful fiber-rich carb full of antioxidants, especially sulfur, which supports the production of glutathione in our bodies. This vital chemical composition maintains the integrity of the gut lining, and in Maintenance, reinforces its regeneration. Flaxseed provides additional omega-3s, magnesium, manganese, protein, vitamin E, and healthy fats for a well-rounded home run at mealtime. When my dear friend Crystal asked me to help her make a cauliflower crust that wasn't soggy, I knew just the trick, and with this recipe, it's yours as well.

Making smaller appetizer-sized mini pizza crusts can be a big hit at your next gathering. Crusts can also be cooked ahead of time and frozen. Reheating in the oven is a snap with no loss of the crunchy crust. I have also taken this crust recipe and cooked it in a square pan to make mock croutons for soup or mock crackers for a snack with hummus. If you are adventurous enough to try this out as crackers or croutons, consider baking them a second time after cutting them up, in similar fashion to making biscotti, for that extra crunch.

- 2 (10-ounce) bags frozen cauliflower, thawed (see notes)
- 1 cup almond meal
- 1 cup nondairy cheese, shredded (I like Violife)
- ⅓ cup ground flaxseed
- 2 tablespoons potato starch

- 1 tablespoon dried herbs (garlic and herb, basil, Herbs de Provence, or rosemary)
- 1 tablespoon dried oregano
- 1 teaspoon salt
- Toppings of your choice (see sidebar)

Preheat the oven to 375°F.

Squeeze out all the excess water from the thawed cauliflower—really squeeze it all out. That's the trick! Put the cauliflower in a big bowl, then add the almond meal, cheese, flaxseed, potato starch, dried herbs, oregano, and salt, mix well with your hands, and form a ball. If you need a little water to tighten up the dough, wet your hands slightly and work the dough like you would knead bread until a tight, slightly sticky ball forms. This happens as the ground flaxseed expands.

Lay a piece of parchment paper on top of a pizza pan. Spread your

Pizza Toppings

It is always recommended to parcook most vegetables before adding them to a pizza, so they will brown and caramelize.

- Chopped mushrooms, sliced tomatoes, and fresh basil
- Shaved brussels sprouts, cheese, and chopped fresh rosemary
- Sautéed broccoli, hot sauce and marinara sauce, and dried oregano
- Artichoke hearts, pickled roasted red pepper slices, banana pepper rings, and dried basil and oregano
- Baby spinach, fresh arugula, sliced cherry tomatoes, and sliced kalamata olives
- Baby kale, roasted butternut squash, sliced red onion, sliced black olives, and dairy-free ricotta

dough out and shape it into a pizza crust. A little time and patience are important here because you are not working with gluten. Flatten the dough as evenly as possible, but remember it does not have to be perfect. Cook for 30 minutes, then remove from the oven. Put a new piece of parchment paper on top of the crust, carefully flip it over, and place it back on the pizza pan. Cook for an additional 15 minutes until golden brown.

If you are making an extra crust to freeze or cooling the crust to use later, remove it from the oven and cool it on a wire rack.

If you're ready to make the pizza, add the toppings of your choice to the crust and put it back in the oven, allowing everything to properly heat up for 10 to 15 minutes.

NOTES: You can use freshly riced cauliflower in this recipe, but steam it first and squeeze out the excess water once it has cooled.

You can also thaw the frozen bags of cauliflower in your refrigerator overnight to save time.

QUINOA VEGETABLE SUSHI WITH SPICY CHICKPEA TAHINI SAUCE
MAKES 2 SERVINGS

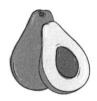

My husband loves to make sushi at home and would live on sushi rice if he could, but I thought of incorporating quinoa to increase the nutritional content of the meal. What you put into the sushi is up to you. I have used sweet potato, purple sweet potato, steamed asparagus, and cooked beets. This is a great way to be creative and use up cooked or raw vegetables. I am a big fan of tahini as it provides so many beneficial functions for our hormones. The spicy combination of chickpeas and the kick of spice is heavenly. We have been putting the extra sauce on everything.

- 2 tablespoons rice vinegar
- 1 tablespoon maple syrup
- 1 teaspoon ground arrowroot

- 1 cup cooked quinoa
- 4 nori sushi sheets
- 1 sweet potato, roasted, cooled, and cut up into several long, thin strips
- 1 avocado, peeled and sliced thin lengthwise
- 1 scallion, cut up into roughly 3-inch strips
- ½ cup Spicy Chickpea Tahini Sauce

SPICY CHICKPEA TAHINI SAUCE:

- 1 cup cooked chickpeas (if canned, drain and rinse well)
- ¼ to ½ cup water
- 2 tablespoons tahini
- 2 tablespoons rice vinegar
- 1 tablespoon sweet chili sauce, sriracha, or other hot sauce

In a small bowl combine the rice vinegar, maple syrup, and arrowroot. Add the quinoa and stir well. Set the mixture aside to cool.

Wrap your sushi mat in plastic wrap and lay it flat on the counter. A sushi mat is a woven bamboo mat; they have been used for centuries in the art of making sushi rolls. Don't fret if you do not own a sushi mat. A simple thick kitchen towel can take the place of a mat. If using a towel, lay plastic wrap on top of it before you begin.

Place the nori sheet smooth side down on the mat. Spoon about ⅓ cup of cooled quinoa onto the entire piece of nori. Use your fingers to cover the nori with the quinoa and gently press it down to distribute it evenly, leaving a 1-inch border at the top and bottom edges. Layer one-quarter of your vegetable strips (sweet potato, avocado, scallion) over the quinoa.

From the bottom, lift the edge and roll the sheet over the vegetables, tucking as you go and rolling as tightly as you can. When you get to the end, wet the edge with water and seal the roll. To cut the roll into pieces, use a sharp knife dipped in water.

To make the Spicy Chickpea Tahini Sauce, put all the ingredients in a high-speed blender or blender cup and blend until well combined. Start with ¼ cup water and add in more as needed to achieve a thick, creamy consistency. Serve with your sushi.

NOTE: The recipe makes about one cup of sauce, which is more than is needed for the bowls, but it is delicious on everything from roasted vegetables to Quinoa Vegetable Sushi and beyond. Keep the sauce in a mason jar in the fridge and use it within a week.

VEGETABLE ENCHILADAS
MAKES 4 LARGE OR 8 SMALL ENCHILADAS

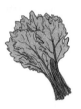

There is no better way to use up summer squash than in a creative, healthy, and delicious recipe everyone will enjoy! If you do not have some of the vegetables listed, chop up what you do have and make it work. Serve with a crispy fresh side salad for a complete meal.

If you double up on the filling, you can use it for quesadillas later. It would also make for a great addition to a Mexican-inspired lasagna (see Green Lentil Lasagna) or a quinoa bowl (see Mexican Rice Bowls). Getting creative with plant-based options builds confidence in so many delicious ways!

- 2 tablespoons olive, coconut, or avocado oil, plus more for greasing pans
- 1 (15-ounce) jar red or green mild enchilada sauce, divided
- 2 garlic cloves, chopped
- ½ onion, chopped
- 3 carrots, grated
- 1 medium zucchini, grated
- 3 cups sautéed Swiss chard, dandelion greens, or any soft greens of your choice, roughly chopped
- 2 tablespoons Taco Seasoning
- 1 (15-ounce) jar mild salsa
- 1 (15-ounce) can refried beans or pinto or black beans, drained and rinsed
- 4 large or 8 small gluten-free tortillas (I like Food for Life, 365, or Siete)
- Nondairy cheese, shredded (I like Violife, optional)
- Optional toppings: chopped cilantro, diced avocados

Preheat the oven to 350°F. Lightly coat the bottom of a large heatproof dish with oil (pump sprays work well too). Pour in about ¼ cup of the enchilada sauce to lightly coat the bottom. Set aside.

Put 2 tablespoons oil in a large pan and sauté the garlic and onion over medium-high heat for several minutes. Add the carrots, zucchini, and baby spinach and continue cooking for 5 to 10 minutes, stirring constantly. Add the Taco Seasoning, salsa, and beans. Remove from the heat and mix well, breaking up the refried beans and thoroughly incorporating all the ingredients.

Put a dash of oil and one tortilla in a frying pan. Warm the tortilla over medium heat for 1 minute and then flip it over and cook for another minute. Repeat with the remaining tortillas.

Now fill the tortillas. This is not a step you want to take your time with. Gluten-free tortillas are not as pliable and need to be warm to work with. Place a tortilla flat on a cutting board and add the filling. If you are making 4 large enchiladas, use about ½ cup filling per tortilla. If you are making 8 smaller enchiladas, use about ¼ to ⅓ cup per tortilla. Top the filling with some shredded cheese (if using), and roll up the tortilla. Place the enchilada fold side down in the prepared dish. Pour the remaining enchilada sauce over the rolled enchiladas and top with some extra shredded cheese, if you like.

Bake in the oven for 25 minutes until bubbly and golden brown. Add the optional toppings of your choice and serve.

NOTE: If you have more filling than you need for one meal, store the leftovers in a freezer-safe container and keep for future use. Baked enchiladas are a snap to reheat on low heat in the oven.

ZESTY BAKED CAULIFLOWER BITES
YIELD VARIES

I say this makes a great side dish, but then I end up eating these delicious savory bites as a meal. I've also used them to top Buddha Bowls. My favorite bowl is quinoa, sautéed Swiss chard, red pepper hummus, and these cauliflower bites. Or use them to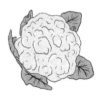

complement a delicious salad or slaw. Either way, be creative and have fun; this is a keeper that you'll often incorporate into mealtime.

- ½ cup water
- ½ cup hot sauce (see note, I like Siete, Red Clay, and Primal Kitchen)
- ¼ cup nutritional yeast
- 2 tablespoons rice or almond flour
- 2 tablespoons tahini or other nut butter
- 2 teaspoons dried herbs (garlic and herb, oregano blend, or another of your choice)
- 1 large head cauliflower, broken up into bite-size pieces

Preheat the oven to 375°F. Line a baking sheet with parchment paper.

In a large bowl, combine the water, hot sauce, nutritional yeast, rice flour, tahini, and dried herbs. Add the cauliflower pieces and toss to evenly coat the cauliflower.

Place the bites 1 inch apart on the prepared baking sheet. Bake for 30 minutes until they look well glazed and golden brown.

NOTE: You can substitute a milder sauce, such as a teriyaki or curry-based sauce, if hot is unappealing to you.

PRESSURE COOKER BEANS

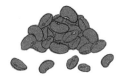

There is such a noticeable difference in taste between canned and home-cooked beans. If you haven't given them a try, using an Instant Pot can be a game changer when it comes to saving money by making fresh beans. (But don't stress if you can't make fresh every time; canned is fine—look for BPA-free cans and rinse the beans well.)

Beans fall into a category of high-protein foods called legumes. Incorporating this plant-based powerhouse into meals provides a source of all nine essential amino acids. In addition, beans are rich in polyphenols and lower in calories and fat compared to animal protein sources.

I recommend rinsing and then soaking the beans overnight, which will remove any potential contaminants, reduce the cooking time, improve the texture, enhance the nutritional value, and give you fewer beans that split open or burst in the cooking process.

Please see the reference chart for bean cooking times. You can try them in any recipes that call for beans, such as Zucchini Noodle Chickpea Salad or homemade Sweet Onion and White Bean Dip. Consider if you will be cooking the beans again after the Instant Pot cooking process, such as in Black Bean Soup. In that case, cut the cooking time by about 5 minutes, so you achieve a more al dente bean.

- The water-to-bean ratio in the pressure cooker is 4 cups water to 1 cup beans.
- To avoid foaming, do not overfill the Instant Pot, and add

Bean Cooking Times

Soaked:

Black	10 to 15 minutes
Black-eyed peas	5 to 10 minutes
Cannellini	0 to 15 minutes
Chickpea (garbanzo)	15 to 20 minutes
Kidney/pinto	10 to 15 minutes
Split peas/lentils	Do not need soaking

Unsoaked:

Black	22 to 27 minutes
Black-eyed peas	10 to 15 minutes
Cannellini	30 to 35 minutes
Chickpea (garbanzo)	35 to 40 minutes
Kidney/pinto	25 to 30 minutes
Split peas	5 to 10 minutes
Lentils	12 to 17 minutes

1 tablespoon olive oil and 1 tablespoon sea salt for every 4 cups water. For reference, the water capacity of most Instant Pots is 8 cups.

- The beans will cook on high pressure. After cooking, you can manually release the steam or, for best quality results, simply wait for the natural release.
- Drain and rinse your cooked beans well in a colander. Save any extra beans for another time by cooling them (use a baking sheet and spread out the beans to cool completely) before storing, whether that's in your refrigerator or freezer.

FLAX-CARROT MOCK FLATBREADS
MAKES 12 (5-INCH) BREADS

What to do with all that carrot pulp after juicing? This recipe was born from trying to use what was being tossed, as I dislike throwing anything away that may have another use. At times, I composted most of this pulp, but I wanted to come up with another way to enjoy the fiber that gets removed by juicing. The result offers a great source of omega-3s as well as beta-carotene and medicinal herbs.

I have used the finished product as a mock bread for an open-faced sandwich (hummus, avocado, tomato, and sprouts) or as the base of a personal pizza. You can get very creative here. Break the rounds apart, toast them more (or dehydrate), and enjoy them as crackers.

- 2 tablespoons olive, coconut, or avocado oil
- 1½ cups flax meal or ground flaxseed
- ½ cup hemp hearts
- 1 cup water
- 4 to 5 cups carrot pulp (see notes)
- 1 teaspoon salt
- 2 tablespoons fresh herbs (parsley, chopped rosemary, basil, or whatever you prefer)
- 2 tablespoons dried herb blend (Italian blend, chimichurri, basil, dill, or cilantro)

Preheat the oven to 350°F. Line a large baking sheet with parchment paper and coat lightly with the oil (pump sprays work well too).

In a large bowl, mix the flax meal, hemp hearts, and water together. Let sit for about 5 minutes. Add in the pulp, salt, fresh herbs, and herb blend and mix thoroughly with your hands. You want the mixture to hold together well.

Use a handful of mixture to form ½-inch thick patties that are about 5 inches in diameter. If the patties are falling apart, the mixture is too dry and you may need to add a bit of water.

Place the patties close together on the prepared baking sheet. You should be able to fit six on each sheet. Sprinkle the tops with additional herbs if you like.

Bake for 30 minutes. Carefully flip each patty and bake for an additional 30 minutes. Refrigerate leftovers and toast to crisp before serving. If freezing, defrost and toast before consuming.

NOTES: You can supplement the carrot pulp with other juiced vegetable pulp such as beet, spinach, celery, ginger, and turmeric, but the majority should be carrot pulp.

Some juicers extract better than others, so if you are lucky enough to have a great juicer, your pulp will be super dry, which means you may need a little more liquid when you mix everything together.

SALADS

ZUCCHINI NOODLE CHICKPEA SALAD
MAKES 2 SERVINGS

Zoodles are all the rage as an alternative to regular pasta. This colorful, hearty salad is refreshing, nutrient dense, and a quick and easy way to make mealtime fun.

- 2 to 3 medium zucchinis, spiralized (see note)
- Handful of baby arugula
- ¼ cup tart cherries, halved
- ½ cup chickpeas
- ¼ cup fresh basil leaves, thinly sliced

DRESSING:

- Juice from 1 orange
- ½ teaspoon fresh ginger, grated
- ½ shallot, thinly sliced
- 3 tablespoons quality olive oil
- 1 teaspoon honey
- 1 teaspoon dried herb blend (chimichurri, lemon and pepper, or garlic and herb)
- ½ teaspoon Dijon mustard

In a large bowl, combine the zucchini, baby arugula, cherries, and chickpeas.

To make the dressing, put all the dressing ingredients in a small bowl or mason jar and whisk or shake until well combined.

Pour half the dressing over the salad and mix lightly to dress. Garnish with basil. Serve immediately. Season with salt and pepper to taste. Store the rest of the dressing in a mason jar in the fridge for up to a week.

NOTE: If using fresh squash, spiralize, and then lay the spirals flat on a tray lined with paper towels. Lightly salt the spirals and let them sweat for 5 to 10 minutes. Use the paper towels to blot excess moisture away. Now you will have super dry noodles that will be extra crunchy and not release excess water that would compromise this delicious salad. You can also use prepackaged 10- to 12-ounce frozen zoodles, which you'll need to defrost. I recommend laying them on a kitchen towel or paper towels prior to defrosting, as they may get very wet.

GREEK QUINOA SALAD
MAKES 4 SERVINGS

This flavorful fiber-rich salad is great as a side dish or complete meal. The addition of quinoa brings a hearty, nutritious element along with fresh flavors and a zippy Greek vinaigrette.

- 2 cups cooked quinoa
- 1 cup grilled vegetables of choice (eggplant, squash, sweet potato)
- 1 medium cucumber, chopped
- 2 tomatoes, chopped, or 1 cup grape tomatoes, halved
- ½ cup kalamata olives, pitted
- ¼ red onion, or 1 medium or large shallot, diced
- ½ cup nondairy feta crumbles (I like Violife)

DRESSING:

- Juice of 2 medium lemons (about ¼ cup)

- ¼ cup olive oil
- 2 tablespoons fresh oregano, chopped
- 2 tablespoons fresh mint, chopped
- 2 tablespoons fresh parsley, chopped

In a large bowl, combine the quinoa, grilled vegetables, cucumber, tomatoes, olives, red onion, and feta.

To make the dressing, put all the dressing ingredients in a small bowl or mason jar and whisk or shake until well combined.

Pour the dressing over the salad and mix lightly to dress. Separate the salad into four bowls and serve immediately. Season with salt and pepper to taste.

FRENCH GREEN LENTIL SALAD
MAKES 3 SERVINGS

French green lentils hold up beautifully in salads and provide a wonderful earthy and slightly peppery flavor that is worth trying out. They also contain more protein than standard green lentils, which are a little milder. Substitute green or brown lentils if needed; either way, you will fall in love with the delicious flavors in this salad.

- 3 cups water or vegetable broth (or a mix)
- 1 cup French green lentils
- ½ cup cooked quinoa
- 1 shallot, diced
- ¼ cup Simple Salad Vinaigrette
- 2 cups fresh arugula
- ¾ cup hummus
- ⅓ cup nondairy feta (I like Violife)
- 6 sun-dried tomatoes, chopped

In a medium saucepan, bring the water and lentils to a boil. Simmer for 15 to 20 minutes until tender. Drain.

Mix the lentils with the quinoa and shallot. Add the Simple Salad Vinaigrette and mix lightly to combine.

Layer each bowl with the arugula, lentil mixture, hummus, and sun-dried tomatoes. Season with salt and pepper to taste. Serve immediately.

CHOPPED KALE SALAD
MAKES 2 SERVINGS

Kale is a dark, leafy green superfood from the cabbage family and is respected for containing an array of nutrients like vitamins A, C, and K, folate, omega-3s, and a handful of impressive minerals.

- 2 cups butternut squash, cut into 1-inch cubes (see note)
- 2 tablespoons olive, coconut, or avocado oil
- 2 shallots, chopped
- 1 bunch of Tuscan kale (a.k.a. dinosaur or lacinato), thinly sliced or chopped (use a knife or food processor)
- ½ cup Simple Salad Vinaigrette
- 1 mango, diced
- ¼ cup pumpkin seeds, toasted
- 1 avocado, diced

Preheat the oven to 350°F. Line a roasting pan with parchment paper. Place the butternut squash on the prepared roasting pan and drizzle with oil (pump sprays work well too). Roast for 25 minutes. Take the pan out of the oven and add the shallots. Cook for an additional 10 minutes until golden brown and the butternut squash edges are starting to caramelize.

When the squash is done, combine the kale and Simple Salad Vinaigrette in a medium bowl and rub the kale thoroughly with your hands to soften it up. Fold in the mango, pumpkin seeds, and avocado. Garnish with the roasted squash and crispy shallots. Season with salt and pepper to taste. Serve immediately.

NOTE: You can save time and purchase packages of fresh, pre-chopped butternut squash. You can also use any leftover roasted vegetables for this recipe; just reheat them in a sauté pan with the shallots.

JICAMA, CUCUMBER, AND CHICKPEA SALAD
MAKES 4 SERVINGS

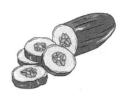

Jicama is a deliciously crunchy and refreshing vegetable that stands up well to all the flavors in this salad. Jicama is packed with nutrients, high in antioxidants, easy on the gut, and good for beneficial bacteria. Look for the vegetable to be about the size of a softball and free of blemishes. The flesh is a beautiful white color once peeled.

- 1 jicama, peeled and shredded
- 2 English cucumbers, diced
- 2 (15-ounce) cans chickpeas, well rinsed, or 3½ cups home-cooked
- 1 shallot, chopped
- 1 mango, diced
- 1 avocado, diced
- ¼ cup pumpkin seeds, roasted

VINAIGRETTE:

- ⅓ cup rice, apple cider, or coconut vinegar
- ¼ cup lime juice
- 1 teaspoon Dijon mustard
- 3 tablespoons olive oil
- 2 tablespoons fresh cilantro, chopped
- 2 tablespoons fresh basil, chopped
- 1 tablespoon fresh oregano, chopped

In a large bowl, combine the jicama, cucumbers, chickpeas, shallot, mango, and avocado.

To make the vinaigrette, put all the vinaigrette ingredients in a small bowl or mason jar and whisk or shake until well combined.

Pour the vinaigrette over the salad and mix lightly to dress. Season with salt and pepper to taste. Garnish with pumpkin seeds and serve.

BUCKWHEAT RAMEN NOODLE AND BOK CHOY SALAD
MAKES 3 SERVINGS

This dish is a favorite in my family. We cannot get enough of this, especially in warmer weather. Bok choy contains many essential minerals, vitamins, and antioxidants. Snap peas are low in calories but pack a punch with fiber, vitamins C and K, and folate. The ramen buckwheat is a delicious alternative to regular pasta and is linked to cancer prevention and better regulation of blood sugar and inflammatory responses.

- 2 packs (about 5 ounces) buckwheat ramen noodles (see notes)
- 1 bunch baby bok choy, thinly sliced
- 6 stalks asparagus, blanched and cut into ½-inch lengths
- 1 red bell pepper, thinly sliced
- 1 carrot, shredded
- 1 cup sugar snap peas, trimmed and julienned (see notes)
- ¼ cup fresh basil, thinly sliced
- ¼ cup fresh cilantro, roughly chopped
- Optional toppings: roasted pumpkin, sesame, or sunflower seeds; lime wedges; thinly sliced avocado; chopped cilantro; chopped scallions

DRESSING:

- ¼ cup coconut or rice vinegar
- ¼ cup coconut aminos
- 2 tablespoons tahini
- 1 tablespoon olive, coconut, or avocado oil
- 1 teaspoon pure maple syrup
- ½ teaspoon fresh ginger, grated
- ½ teaspoon lime zest
- Juice of 1 lime (about 3 to 4 tablespoons)

Cook the noodles according to the package directions and rinse with cool water to keep them from sticking together. Put the noodles in a big bowl. Add the bok choy, asparagus, bell pepper, carrot, snap peas, basil, and cilantro and mix gently. Set aside.

To make the dressing, put all the ingredients in a small bowl or mason jar and whisk or shake until well combined.

Pour the dressing over the salad and mix lightly to dress. Season with salt and pepper to taste. Serve with the toppings of your choice and enjoy.

NOTES: Look for 100 percent buckwheat noodles. King Soba brand is organic and has a 9.8-ounce package that's enough for 4 servings. There are also soup mixes (Lotus Foods, Big Green, and Onetang) with millet and brown rice noodles; just omit the soup seasoning packet and use the noodles.

Wondering how to trim a snap pea? It's important because eating a snap pea with the vein intact is unpleasant and hard to chew. The tip or string should be dangling and attached to the concave side of the shell. Use a small paring knife to grab the string and pull along the side. It will come off easily. Once you pull off the first tip, pull the second tip in the opposite direction and discard.

BUCKWHEAT SOBA NOODLE SALAD
MAKES 4 SERVINGS

This is a great dinner salad, and this recipe makes enough leftovers for lunch the next day. This salad can be served with warm noodles and dressing or as a cold salad on a hot summer day. Either way, it's bursting with flavor and nutrients.

- 8 ounces buckwheat soba noodles
- 4 cups romaine, chopped, or Bibb lettuce
- ¾ cup snow peas or green peas, trimmed and julienned
- 1 small head radicchio, chopped
- ¼ red onion, chopped
- 2 carrots, shredded
- 4 scallions, chopped

- Optional toppings: sliced or cubed avocado, white sesame
  seeds, chopped cilantro

DRESSING:

- ½ cup Chef Lisa DeNiear's Cilantro-Lime Sauce
- 2 tablespoons maple syrup
- 1 tablespoon tahini
- 1 tablespoon rice or coconut vinegar

Bring a large pot of salted water to a boil. Add the soba noodles and cook for 4 minutes over medium-high heat. Start testing your noodles after 4 minutes and look for something close to al dente. Do not over-cook the noodles as they will become gummy. Drain and rinse under cool water. Put the noodles in a medium bowl and set aside.

In a large bowl, combine the lettuce, snow peas, radicchio, red onion, carrots, and scallions.

To make the dressing, put all the dressing ingredients in a small bowl or mason jar and whisk or shake until well combined. Add half the dressing to the noodles and fold in. Set aside.

Layer each plate with the lettuce combination, cooled noodles (or if you are having this as a warm dish, reheated noodles), and the toppings of your choice. Divide the remaining dressing between each plate, season with salt and pepper to taste, and serve immediately.

SHAVED BRUSSELS SPROUT SALAD WITH LEMON-SHALLOT VINAIGRETTE
MAKES 4 TO 6 SIDE SERVINGS

Brussels sprouts are a member of the cabbage family. They are touted as a superfood with an impressive source of vitamins C and K and fiber. They are a prebiotic and sulfur-rich food. This earns brussels sprouts kudos as a considerable 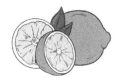 *source of disease-fighting antioxidants. Radishes are a root vegetable rich in antioxidants and the minerals calcium and potassium. It is the vegetable of choice for improved blood flow! White watermelon seeds are an incredible source of the much-needed nutrient magnesium. This underrated anti-inflammatory nutrient contributes to bone health, fights depression, and protects against type 2 diabetes and high blood pressure. The best part of this salad is that it holds up for days in the refrigerator. Give it a good stir to wake up all the delicious flavors and enjoy!*

- 16 ounces brussels sprouts, cleaned (remove any browned leaves) and bottoms cut off
- 1 cup radishes, sliced
- 1 (15-ounce) can chickpeas, well rinsed, or 1½ cups home-cooked
- 1 yellow bell pepper, diced
- ¼ cup white watermelon, pumpkin, or sunflower seeds, toasted
- ¼ cup dried cherries or cranberries, sliced

VINAIGRETTE:

- ⅓ cup lemon juice
- ¼ cup olive oil
- 1 shallot, chopped
- ¼ cup fresh parsley, chopped
- 1 tablespoon fresh tarragon, chopped
- 1 tablespoon Dijon mustard
- 1 teaspoon maple syrup
- ½ teaspoon lemon zest

Pulse the brussels sprouts in a food processor until they are finely shaved or use the slicing attachment. You can also use a mandolin or sharp knife.

In a large bowl, combine the brussels sprouts, radishes, chickpeas, bell pepper, watermelon seeds, and cherries.

To make the vinaigrette, put all the vinaigrette ingredients in a small bowl or mason jar and whisk or shake until well combined.

Add the vinaigrette to the salad, toss well, season with salt and pepper to taste, and serve.

THAI CHOPPED SALAD
MAKES 4 TO 6 SIDE SERVINGS

This delicious and diverse salad will keep for several days in the refrigerator. It is bright, fresh, and offers a well-rounded plate full of nutrients.

- 3 cups kale, shredded and chopped (lacinato or curly)
- 1 cup napa cabbage, shredded
- 1 cup fresh or frozen peas, blanched
- 3 large carrots, shredded
- 2 scallions, thinly sliced
- 1 red bell pepper, thinly sliced
- 1 yellow bell pepper, thinly sliced
- 1 avocado, diced
- 1 mango, diced
- ½ cup cashews or almonds, chopped (optional)

VINAIGRETTE:

- ¼ cup olive oil
- 1 tablespoon chili garlic sauce (see note)
- ¼ cup water
- 2 tablespoons honey or maple syrup
- 1 tablespoon fresh ginger, grated
- 2 tablespoons rice vinegar
- 1 tablespoon sesame oil
- ¼ cup coconut aminos
- 1 lime, zested and juiced
- 1 teaspoon fresh mint, chopped
- 1 tablespoon fresh basil, chopped
- 1 tablespoon fresh cilantro, chopped

In a large bowl, combine the kale, cabbage, peas, carrots, scallions, and bell peppers.

To make the vinaigrette, put all the vinaigrette ingredients in a small bowl or mason jar and whisk or shake until well combined.

Add about half the dressing to the salad and massage it into the greens for a minute or two. Fold in the avocado, mango, and nuts (if using). Taste and add the remaining vinaigrette as needed. Season with salt and pepper to taste.

NOTE: You can find chili garlic paste in the Asian section of the grocery store. It is great for adding a kick of spice to many sauces, soups, and dressings.

FENNEL COLESLAW WITH GRAPEFRUIT DRESSING
MAKES 4 TO 5 SERVINGS

Fennel is an excellent source of calcium and dietary fiber, while cabbage is a member of the cruciferous family and is rich in antioxidants. Cabbage also has high levels of minerals such as calcium, iron, iodine, potassium, sulfur, and phosphorus. In the vitamin department, it is loaded: vitamins A, B_1, B_2, B_6, C, E, and K and folic acid.

Both cabbage and fennel are super low in calories. The combination of additional ingredients is complementary and so wonderfully delicious, you may find yourself making this salad again and again.

- 1½ cups cabbage, finely shredded, or 1 package coleslaw mix, finely chopped (see notes)
- 1 fennel bulb, shredded or grated
- 2 carrots, shredded or grated
- 1 red bell pepper, chopped
- 1 zucchini, shredded or grated
- 1 avocado, diced
- 1 mango, diced
- ¼ cup slivered almonds
- Handful of fresh cilantro, chopped

DRESSING:

- Juice of 2 grapefruits (about 1½ cups)
- ¼ cup lemon juice

- ½ cup olive oil
- 1 shallot, chopped
- 5 pickled jalapeños
- 1 tablespoon Dijon mustard
- ¼ cup white wine vinegar
- 1 tablespoon dried herb blend (garlic and herb, tarragon, or lemon pepper)

In a large bowl, combine the cabbage, fennel, carrots, bell pepper, and zucchini.

To make the dressing, put all the dressing ingredients in a high-speed blender or food processor and blend until well combined and smooth.

Add half the dressing to the cabbage mixture and massage it into the coleslaw with your hands or a spoon. Fold in the avocado and mango. Season with salt and pepper to taste. Garnish with almonds and cilantro, and serve with the rest of the dressing.

NOTES: For the cabbage or coleslaw, I recommend using a packaged mix and pulsing it several times in a food processor.

If you do not plan on serving the entire salad, save the dressing separate from the greens.

SOUPS

GOLDEN BEET GAZPACHO
MAKES 4 SERVINGS

This is a vibrant, delicious way to enjoy golden beets. Golden beets are slightly sweeter than red beets, but both are powerhouses of essential minerals and vitamins. Beets boost whole-body detoxification and aid in supporting the immune system.

- 6 to 7 small or 4 to 5 medium golden beets, peeled, roughly cut, and boiled until tender (reserve 2 cups of cooking water)
- 2 English cucumbers, peeled, seeded, and roughly chopped
- 2 cloves Roasted Garlic (see note)
- 1 shallot, chopped
- ¼ cup lemon juice
- 2 tablespoons olive oil
- 1 tablespoon sherry vinegar
- Optional garnishes: diced cooked golden beets, diced avocado, pickled red onion, lemon juice

Blend the beets, cucumbers, garlic, shallot, lemon juice, olive oil, and sherry vinegar in a high-speed blender or food processor until completely smooth. I like thick gazpacho, but if you prefer it thinner, add some of the saved beet water and blend. Season with salt to taste.

Chill for at least an hour before adding the garnishes of your choice and serving.

NOTE: You can also use raw garlic; I prefer roasted as it has a more mellow flavor.

DOCTORED-UP BEAN SOUP MIXES
MAKES 10 TO 12 SERVINGS

Moments occur all too often in our lives when time is simply not on our side. When trying to keep up with a healthier lifestyle, putting something together without a lot of guesswork is key, and that's where this recipe comes into play. The most important aspect of using a pre-made bean soup mix is, of course, label reading. Look at the packaging and make sure it is non-GMO certified with no added salt or artificial ingredients.

- 2 tablespoons olive oil
- 1 onion, diced
- 4 to 5 celery stalks, diced
- 3 large carrots, roughly chopped
- 1 package dried-bean soup mix (Frontier, Bob's Red Mill)
- 12 cups water or vegetable broth (see notes)
- 1 (16-ounce) package frozen butternut squash, diced (see notes)
- Bouquet garni of fresh rosemary, thyme, and sage
- ½ cup cooked gluten-free elbow pasta (see notes)

Put the oil, onion, celery, and carrots in a large stockpot and sauté over medium-high heat, stirring occasionally, for 10 minutes. Stir in the soup mix, its herb packet (if using, see notes), and water. Add the butternut squash and bouquet garni, stir, cover, and bring to a boil. Turn the heat down and simmer, still covered, for 45 minutes.

Remove from the heat and add the pasta. Let it sit for 10 minutes; it should become thick like a stew. You can thin it out with broth for more of a soup consistency, if you like. Remove the bouquet garni, season with salt and pepper to taste, and serve.

NOTES: If the added packet of seasonings and sodium is higher than 10 percent of your daily recommended allowance, throw it away (or just use half) and use an organic vegetable broth in its place. If you are using the packet, just use water.

If you don't have frozen butternut squash, any type of frozen root vegetables will work. This is a good opportunity to clean out your freezer! You can also substitute 2 fresh diced sweet potatoes.

For the gluten-free pasta, I love Trader Joe's brown rice and quinoa mini elbow pasta, but anything similar will work. Chickapea brand shells hold up well in soups and stews also. The pasta should be cooked just shy of al dente before adding it to the soup, so cut about 2 minutes from the manufacturer's recommended cooking time for best results.

BLACK BEAN SOUP
MAKES 6 SERVINGS

This simple, hearty soup is loaded with the soluble fiber our bodies need. Soluble fiber expands in our stomachs when consumed and sends satiety signals to our brains, letting us know we are full. The insoluble fiber found in vegetables aids in proper digestion. Both fibers are important for keeping your insulin levels balanced and preventing the impulse to snack in between meals. Pair with a side salad for a perfect meal.

- 2 tablespoons olive, coconut, or avocado oil
- 1 onion, diced
- 3 carrots, diced
- 3 celery stalks, diced
- 4 garlic cloves, finely chopped (optional)
- 1 serrano or jalapeño pepper, finely diced (optional)
- 1 tablespoon ground cumin
- 2 (15-ounce) cans black beans, well rinsed, or 4 cups home-cooked
- 1 (8-ounce) can diced tomatoes
- 1 cup canned pumpkin
- 4 to 5 cups vegetable broth
- Handful of fresh parsley, chopped
- Handful of fresh cilantro, chopped
- Avocado, diced (optional)

Put the oil, onion, carrots, celery, garlic, serrano pepper, and cumin in a large stockpot and cook over medium heat for several minutes, stirring occasionally. Stir in the black beans, tomatoes, pumpkin, and vegetable broth and bring to a gentle boil. Cover and simmer for 30 to 40 minutes. Stir in the fresh herbs. Remove from the heat, and let sit for at least 10 minutes.

Use an immersion blender to blend about half the soup to thicken as desired. You can also blend about half the soup in small batches in a high-speed blender once the soup has slightly cooled. Season with salt and pepper to taste. Serve hot with avocado on top (if using). Leftovers can be frozen for another meal.

BLACK LENTIL MINESTRONE
MAKES 6 TO 8 SERVINGS

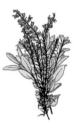

Black lentils are a great source of protein, fiber, potassium, magnesium, iron, folate, and zinc. They are the most nutritious member of the lentil family and hold up well in soups.

Most times when I make soup, I freeze an extra quart. There have been many occasions when those forgotten soups were lifesavers, such as on a hectic evening or when a friend was sick or in need of a meal. Then there are the moments when I have taken two different soups from the freezer and put them together for a surprisingly fabulous meal.

- 3 tablespoons olive, coconut, or avocado oil
- 1 red onion, chopped
- 1 large or 2 small fennel bulbs, roughly chopped (reserve fronds)
- 3 large carrots, roughly chopped
- 2 cups fresh or frozen butternut squash, roughly chopped (see notes)
- 8 stalks asparagus, roughly chopped
- Bouquet garni of fresh parsley, rosemary, and thyme
- 1½ cups black lentils (beluga or regular)
- 4 to 6 cups vegetable broth

- 1 (15-ounce) can diced tomatoes
- 2 cups gluten-free pasta shells or other small pasta (see notes)
- Optional toppings: parsley, basil, fennel fronds

Put the oil, onion, fennel, and carrots in a large stockpot and sauté over medium heat for about 10 minutes, stirring frequently. Add the butternut squash and asparagus and stir for several minutes. Add the bouquet garni and stir gently for 2 more minutes. Stir in the lentils and 4 cups of the broth, cover, and simmer for about 20 minutes. Stir in the tomatoes (and their liquid) and the pasta shells, re-cover, and continue to simmer for an additional 15 to 20 minutes. If you find that the soup is too thick, add the remaining 2 cups broth. The soup will also thicken as it cools.

Season with salt and pepper to taste and add your toppings of choice. Serve immediately.

NOTES: If you don't have butternut squash, any 16-ounce bag of frozen root vegetables will work. This is a good opportunity to clean out your freezer! You can also substitute 2 fresh diced sweet potatoes.

For the pasta shells, I like 365 or Chickapea brand shells because they hold up nicely in soup.

HEALTHFUL VEGETABLE STEW
MAKES 6 TO 8 SERVINGS

This is hands down one of my favorite vegetable stews made with black-eyed peas. It's a perfect maintenance recipe where healthy plant-based ingredients remain center stage.

- ¼ cup olive oil, plus extra to serve
- 1 yellow onion, chopped
- 4 to 5 celery stalks, chopped
- 4 to 5 large carrots, peeled and chopped
- 1 large or 2 small fennel bulbs, trimmed, halved, and sliced into thin strips
- 2 cloves Roasted Garlic

- 4 cups frozen black-eyed peas, or 2 (15-ounce) cans, well rinsed (see notes)
- 2 cups diced fresh or frozen butternut squash (see notes)
- 2 sweet or white potatoes, diced
- 2 tomatoes, diced, or 1 (15-ounce) can diced tomatoes
- 2 tablespoons tomato paste
- 2 to 3 bay leaves
- ⅛ teaspoon salt
- 4 cups vegetable broth
- 2 to 4 cups water
- 1 cup kale, roughly chopped
- 1 cup spinach, roughly chopped
- ½ cup fresh dill, chopped
- Lemon wedges

Heat the olive oil in a large stockpot over medium heat. Add the onion, celery, carrots, and fennel and sauté for about 10 minutes, stirring often. Add the garlic, peas, butternut squash, potatoes, tomatoes, and tomato paste. Work the tomato paste in evenly among the other ingredients. Add the bay leaves, salt, vegetable broth, and enough extra water to cover the vegetables. Bring the ingredients to a boil, cover, and simmer slowly for 40 minutes.

Stir in the kale, spinach, and dill. Cook for another 10 minutes and season with extra salt and pepper to taste.

To serve, drizzle with a dash of olive oil and a squeeze of fresh lemon juice to enhance the overall flavor.

NOTES: If you prefer to use fresh black-eyed peas, soak 2 cups of dried beans in a large pot filled with cool water. Boil for 1 minute and remove from the heat. Set aside and soak for 1 hour before starting the stew. Rinse and drain the peas before adding them to the stew. In addition, add another 10 minutes to the simmer time of the stew. If the liquid level gets too low, add more water or broth (taste the stew to see which you think would be better). The beans should be tender, but not mushy.

If you don't have butternut squash, any 16-ounce bag of frozen root vegetables will work. This is a good opportunity to clean out your freezer!

GREEN CURRY BUTTERNUT SQUASH STEW
MAKES 6 SERVINGS

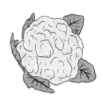

This creamy, flavorful stew is packed with nutritious and anti-inflammatory ingredients. The combination of flavors produces a rich, hearty, and flavorful meal that tastes like you cooked it for hours. You set aside half the veggies at the beginning of the cooking process, then puree the rest to create a smooth yet chunky stew that hits every note for taste and satiety.

- 3 tablespoons olive, coconut, or avocado oil, divided
- 1 tablespoon green curry paste (look for it in the Asian section of your supermarket)
- ¾ cup full-fat unsweetened canned coconut milk, divided
- 1 cup mirepoix (equal amounts diced carrots, celery, and onion, see notes)
- 2 leeks, cleaned and thinly sliced
- 2 garlic cloves, chopped (optional)
- 2 medium butternut squash, peeled and cubed, divided (about 9 cups, see notes)
- 1 head cauliflower, roughly chopped (see notes)
- 1 cup red lentils, divided
- 5 cups vegetable broth, divided
- Lime wedges
- Cilantro, chopped

Heat 1 tablespoon of the oil in a small pot over medium heat, then stir in the curry paste and sauté for 1 minute to release the aromatic flavors. Add ¼ cup of the coconut milk and whisk it into the curry paste. Remove from the heat.

Heat the remaining 2 tablespoons oil in a large stockpot over medium-high heat, then add the mirepoix, leeks, garlic, and about 3 cups of the butternut squash. Cook, stirring occasionally, for 5 minutes. Put half the mixture in a large bowl and set aside.

Add the cauliflower, remaining 6 cups butternut squash, lentils, 4 cups of the broth, and the curry paste mixture to the large stockpot and cook for an additional 5 to 7 minutes, stirring occasionally. Bring to a boil and simmer for 25 minutes.

Remove from the heat and blend with an immersion blender for 2 to 3 minutes until the mixture is roughly pureed. You can also blend a portion of the soup in small batches in a high-speed blender once the soup has slightly cooled. Return the vegetable mixture that you set aside to the pot with the pureed mixture and simmer over low to medium heat for an additional 20 minutes. Stir in the remaining broth ½ cup at a time until the soup reaches your desired consistency. Remove from the heat and stir in the remaining ½ cup coconut milk. Season with salt and pepper to taste.

Garnish with lime wedges and cilantro and serve hot.

NOTES: You can often find prepared mirepoix in the produce section.

The amount of butternut squash does not have to be exact. One 20-ounce package of diced butternut squash is about 5 cups, so you could just use 2 packages. If it's too thick, you can thin it out with more broth. You can substitute broccoli or chopped spinach for the cauliflower—or use a combination of all three!

ROASTED VEGETABLES AND MUSHROOM STEW
MAKES 8 SERVINGS

This soup was the result of my cleaning out the fridge one day. I love mushrooms, especially when sautéed and finished with sherry or cooking wine. This soup is built on the deep flavors of caramelizing the mushrooms with sherry/wine on the stovetop and roasting the vegetables in the oven.

Whole-grain buckwheat is a gluten-free superfood option that is like barley in texture. The benefits of buckwheat shine, as it is a great source of protein, fiber, zinc, magnesium, and folate. In combination with the additional ingredients below, it makes for a hearty, nutritiously rich, and deeply satisfying stew worthy of a cold night in front of a fire.

- 3 tablespoons olive, coconut, or avocado oil, divided
- 1 pound baby portobello mushrooms, halved

- 1 pound shiitake mushrooms, sliced
- 3 shallots, chopped
- ¾ cup cooking sherry or cooking wine
- 1 yellow or Vidalia onion, roughly chopped
- ½ butternut squash, roughly chopped, or 2 cups frozen (see notes)
- 2 russet potatoes, peeled and roughly diced into bite-size pieces
- 4 celery stalks, roughly sliced
- Bouquet garni of 8 to 10 fresh sage leaves and 8 to 10 fresh thyme sprigs (see notes)
- 2 tablespoons basil pesto
- 1 (15-ounce) can butternut squash or sweet potato puree
- 1 (15-ounce) can white beans, drained and rinsed
- 1 (15-ounce) can diced tomatoes
- 4 to 5 cups vegetable broth
- ¾ cup buckwheat groats
- Salt and pepper

Preheat the oven to 375°F. Line a roasting pan with parchment paper and coat it evenly with about 1 tablespoon of the oil (pump sprays work well too).

Coat a cast-iron pan with 2 tablespoons of the oil and heat over medium-high heat. Add the mushrooms and shallots and sauté, stirring attentively, for 10 to 15 minutes. When the mushrooms and shallots start to caramelize, add the sherry and continue to stir. Let the sherry cook off and continue to stir until you have a deep, rich-looking pan of mushrooms. Remove from the heat and set aside.

Evenly spread the onion, butternut squash, potatoes, and celery in the roasting pan. Cook for 20 minutes, then remove the pan and flip the vegetables. Place the bouquet garni on top of the vegetables and return them to the oven for 10 to 15 minutes.

When the vegetables are done, combine the mushroom mixture, roasted vegetables, bouquet garni, pesto, butternut squash puree, beans, tomatoes, and 4 cups of the broth in a large stockpot. Bring the soup to a low boil and cook for 25 minutes. Add the buckwheat groats and cook for an additional 10 minutes. If you would like to thin out the stew, add in the remaining 1 cup vegetable broth. Remove the bouquet garni, season with salt and pepper to taste, and serve immediately.

NOTES: If you don't have butternut squash, any 16-ounce bag of frozen root vegetables will work. This is a good opportunity to clean out your freezer!

If you don't have fresh herbs, substitute dried herbs. Typically, the rule is 3 parts fresh to 1 part dried.

SNACKS AND DESSERTS

CREAMY MOCK COOKIE DOUGH
MAKES 2 SERVINGS

This is a fun and interesting way to use a white sweet potato, which is a wonderful source of vitamin C. Unlike the orange sweet potato, the white version is often used as a base in dessert recipes because it's blander and drier.

- 1½ cups cooked white sweet potato or Japanese white sweet potato, cut into chunks
- 3 Medjool dates, pitted
- 2 to 4 tablespoons oat or coconut milk
- 2 tablespoons sunflower or almond butter
- 1 teaspoon vanilla extract
- ½ teaspoon salt
- ¼ cup mini dark chocolate chips

Start by steaming or boiling the potatoes.

To steam, put about 3 inches of water in a steamer and bring to a boil. Add the potatoes to the steamer tray. Cover and steam for about 15 minutes until tender.

To boil, bring salted water and potatoes to a boil in a large pot. Cook until tender, 10 to 12 minutes.

Let the potatoes cool slightly and then combine them with the dates, milk, sunflower butter, vanilla, and salt in a high-speed blender and blend until smooth and creamy. You will achieve a better consistency if the potatoes are still slightly warm. If the batter is too thick, add more milk to get a creamier consistency.

Fold in the chocolate chips and chill for at least an hour before serving.

VERY BERRY CHIA OATS
MAKES 4 SERVINGS

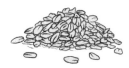

This quick recipe will help you save more time during the rest of the week, but remember that it is a recipe that needs to sit in the fridge overnight. In the morning, you will have the base for a perfect snack to layer with more healthful additions like ground flaxseed, granola, or dried mulberries. This type of meal or snack is great on the go because it can be assembled and transported in a mason jar for convenience.

- ½ cup white chia seeds
- 1 cup rolled or quick oats (see notes)
- ⅓ cup superfood powder (optional, see notes)
- 1½ cups frozen dark cherries, strawberries, blueberries, raspberries, or a combination (see notes)
- 1 banana
- 3 to 4 cups nondairy milk of choice (almond, coconut, oat, or flax), divided

Combine the chia seeds, oats, and superfood powder (if using) in a large bowl. Set aside.

Blend the frozen fruit, banana, and 1 cup of the milk in a high-speed blender or blender cup until well combined.

Combine the wet ingredients with the dry. Add 2 cups of the milk, stirring constantly with a whisk or fork to break up any clumps.

Wait 10 minutes and whisk again. It should be visibly thicker, but not so thick that you cannot move it around. If after the initial 10 minutes it is still too runny, add a handful of chia seeds and stir again. If it's too thick, try thinning it out with a little extra milk.

Cover tightly and put in the fridge to set for at least 6 hours or overnight. The milk should plump up the chia seeds, resulting in a pudding-like consistency.

NOTES: Regular rolled oats offer a chewier texture, while quick oats are smoother.

For the superfood powder, look for pomegranate, acai, or passion fruit or a mixture. Navitas Organics and Sunfood Superfoods are great brands.

For the frozen fruit, look for smoothie starters and berry mixes in the frozen aisle. They are a great way to be creative and save time.

CHIA PUDDING
MAKES 4 SERVINGS

Chia seeds are one of the richest sources of omega-3s available, and they deliver massive amounts of nutrients—fiber, protein, calcium, and magnesium—with very few calories. The phytoestrogens in flax-seed help reduce the frequency of hot flashes. Hempseeds may also help regulate hormonal imbalances and the inflammation associated with menopause. Embrace this superfood.

This type of meal or snack is great on the go because it can be assembled and transported in a mason jar for convenience. Just remember that it needs to set overnight!

- ½ cup white or black chia seeds
- 2 cups nondairy milk of choice (almond, coconut, oat, or flax)

Put the chia seeds and milk in a medium bowl and mix well with a whisk, breaking up any clumps of chia. Wait for 10 minutes and whisk again. It should be visibly thicker, but not so thick that you cannot move it around. If it is too runny, add a handful of chia seeds and stir again. If it's too thick, try thinning it out with a little extra milk.

Cover tightly and put it in the fridge overnight or for at least 3 hours to set. The milk should plump up the chia seeds, resulting in a pudding-like consistency.

Yogurt Parfait

Making a yogurt parfait is all about being creative. It's basically a fun way to layer yogurt and whatever healthy accoutrements (fruit, nuts, seeds, ground flaxseed or hempseed, granola, dried mulberries, or dried fruit) you desire. There are many plant-based yogurts available (see Pantry Must-Haves).

This type of meal or snack is great on the go because it can be assembled and transported in a mason jar for convenience. Parfaits are wonderful fuel for the body and brain when you pick your ingredients wisely. Skip the flavored yogurts and buy plain. You will be surprised how quickly you get used to the lack of added sugar. Add unsweetened dried fruits, and you'll have all the nutrients—protein, fiber, natural sugars, and healthy fats—needed to fuel your body.

Ground flaxseed, chia, and hemp hearts are the quickest and most nutrient-dense addition to a yogurt parfait, smoothie, bowl of cereal, or warm oatmeal breakfast. Our bodies will digest these ground versions better than the whole seeds, which need to expand before delivering nutrients. Seeds are often harder on the digestive tract as well. The diverse use of these superfoods is the best dietary choice you can make for overall health.

You can use bases such as Chia Pudding, Very Berry Chia Oats, Oven-Dried Mulberries, or Simple Granola in addition to some yogurt. Get creative with snacks or mealtime with the following suggestions:

- Chia Pudding with layers of yogurt, fresh fruit, and Simple Granola
- Chia Pudding with layers of yogurt, dried goji berries, and dried mulberries
- Plain yogurt, sliced bananas, fresh blueberries, and hemp hearts
- Plain yogurt, ground flaxseed, fresh applesauce, fresh blackberries, and toasted pumpkin seeds

NOTE: If you would like to add some sweetness, blend a banana into the milk before adding it to the chia seeds. Any fruit will do; try a frozen acai packet or other frozen fruits too. Getting creative is easy once you have mastered the base! Make sure you can stir the pudding and it's not too thick prior to refrigerating it overnight.

SIMPLE GRANOLA
MAKES 4 CUPS

Just a handful of ingredients make up this simple granola. For the most perfect clumpy granola, make sure you press it down into an even layer before it goes into the oven and then again after it comes out. Also, keep in mind the granola will get crunchier as it cools.

- ½ cup maple syrup
- 1 tablespoon vanilla extract
- ½ cup coconut oil, melted
- 4 cups rolled oats
- 1 teaspoon cinnamon
- ¾ teaspoon salt
- 1 cup almonds and pecans, chopped
- 2 cups dried fruit, diced (I like golden raisins and apricots)

Preheat the oven to 325°F. Line a 10 x 10-inch baking pan with parchment paper.

Put the maple syrup and vanilla in a large bowl and whisk to combine. Whisk in the oil. Stir in the oats, cinnamon, salt, and nuts until everything is well coated. You may want to use your hands to mix it well.

Spread the granola mixture out on the prepared baking pan, pressing it down in an even layer. Bake for 35 minutes. Stir the granola halfway through the cooking time to ensure even baking. Take the granola out and mix the dried fruit into the granola. Then cook an additional 10 minutes. It should get nice and golden. The fruit may smell like it is starting to burn, but it is all part of the unique taste!

Remove the granola from the oven, press it down, and let it cool completely before breaking it apart. Store in an airtight container for several weeks or freeze to extend freshness.

OATMEAL RAISIN COOKIES
MAKES ABOUT 2 DOZEN COOKIES

These cookies are the perfect alternative to typical cookies loaded with sugar. The buckwheat cereal boosts fiber, resistant-starch, and high-quality protein.

- 2 tablespoons ground flaxseed
- 1 tablespoon hemp hearts
- 6 tablespoons water
- ⅓ cup maple syrup
- 1 teaspoon vanilla extract
- ⅓ cup coconut oil
- ½ cup oats
- 1 cup buckwheat cereal
- ¾ cup brown or white rice flour
- ½ teaspoon baking powder
- ½ teaspoon baking soda
- 1 teaspoon ground cinnamon
- ¼ teaspoon salt
- ¾ cup raisins

Preheat the oven to 350°F. Line a baking sheet with parchment paper.

In a large bowl, create the flax egg by combining the flaxseed, hemp hearts, and water and letting it sit for 5 minutes. Then, add the maple syrup, vanilla, and oil. Whisk to incorporate and set aside.

In a medium bowl, combine the oats, buckwheat cereal, rice flour, baking powder, baking soda, cinnamon, and salt. Add the dry ingredients to the wet and stir until you get a uniform batter. Fold in the raisins.

Using a large cookie scoop or spoon, place 1-inch balls about 2 inches apart on the parchment paper. Flatten slightly into round disks using a fork or two fingers. Put in the oven and bake for 15 minutes, until slightly browned. Remove from the oven and cool before eating.

JENNIPHER'S GINGERBREAD COOKIES
MAKES 24 COOKIES

A dear client of mine shared this recipe with me as we both love ginger and wanted a healthier snack option. It is my honor to include this indulgence full of warm flavors, omega-3s from the flax, and anti-inflammatory properties from the fresh ginger. With a balance of fiber, protein, and healthy fat, and an array of vitamins and minerals that you will not find with most store-bought impersonators, this is a decadent treat sans guilt.

- ¼ cup maple syrup
- 4 Medjool dates, pitted
- ¼ cup unsweetened applesauce
- 3 tablespoons ground flaxseed
- ¼ cup almond butter
- ⅓ cup molasses
- 2 teaspoons vanilla
- 2 teaspoons lemon juice
- 2 teaspoons fresh ginger, grated
- ½ cup buckwheat flour
- ½ cup brown rice flour
- 1 teaspoon cinnamon
- 1 teaspoon allspice
- 1 tablespoon tapioca starch or flour
- ½ teaspoon baking soda

Preheat the oven to 350°F. Line a baking sheet with parchment paper.

Put the maple syrup, dates, and applesauce in a food processor or high-speed blender and blend or puree for about 30 seconds until you have a thick paste. Put the mixture in a large bowl. Add the flaxseed, almond butter, molasses, vanilla, lemon juice, and ginger and mix well. Let sit for 5 minutes.

Fold in the buckwheat flour, brown rice flour, cinnamon, allspice, tapioca starch, and baking soda and mix until it resembles a thick cookie dough.

Place 1 heaping tablespoon of dough about 2 inches apart on the prepared baking sheet. Bake for 10 minutes until golden brown. As good as they smell fresh out of the oven, I recommend waiting about 5 minutes for the cookies to firm up before enjoying. Store in an airtight container.

CHOCOLATE CHIP CHERRY AND COCONUT BARS
MAKES 15 TO 20 BARS

Coconut oil contains medium-chain unsaturated (good) fats that the body uses to produce energy. It is said to have components with thyroid-stimulating, antiaging, anticancer, and antiviral effects as well as weight loss stimulating properties. Tart cherries, whether in juice form or fresh or dried, have among the highest levels of disease-fighting anti-oxidants. Tart cherries also increase melatonin in the body.

- 3 tablespoons ground flaxseed
- ¼ cup water
- ¼ cup coconut oil, melted
- 1½ cups applesauce
- ⅓ cup maple syrup
- 1 tablespoon vanilla extract
- 1 cup brown or white rice flour
- ½ cup buckwheat cereal
- ¼ cup coconut flour
- 1 teaspoon baking powder
- 1 teaspoon salt
- ¾ cup dark chocolate chips
- ½ cup dried cherries or other dried fruit (blueberries, figs, apricots)

Preheat the oven to 250°F. Line an 8 x 8-inch baking pan with parchment paper.

In a large bowl, create the flax egg by combining the flaxseed and water and letting it sit for 5 minutes. Add the oil, applesauce, maple syrup, and vanilla and mix well with a whisk.

In a small bowl, combine the rice flour, buckwheat cereal, coconut flour, baking powder, and salt. Add the dry ingredients to the wet. Add the chocolate chips and dried cherries and mix well to combine. Spread evenly in the prepared pan. Bake for 20 minutes until golden brown. Wait until slightly cooled to cut and enjoy.

NO-BAKE ENERGY SQUARES
MAKES 35 TO 40 SQUARES

This satiating combination of high fiber, protein, carbohydrates, and healthy fats is the perfect on-the-go (or in the comfort of your home) snack. The squares provide a boost of energy and will leave you full for hours. In addition, these bite-size goodies impress with much-needed iron, magnesium, calcium, vitamin A, B vitamins, and potassium along with antioxidants, bone-strengthening minerals, and omega-3s. They are packed with flavor, anti-inflammatory properties, immune support, and nutrients galore!

- ¼ cup hemp hearts
- ¼ cup ground flaxseed
- ¼ cup chia seeds
- ⅓ cup water
- 20 Medjool dates, pitted
- ⅓ cup dried goji berries
- ¼ cup pumpkin seeds
- 4 dried figs
- ¼ cup cacao nibs
- ¼ cup dark chocolate chips
- 1 teaspoon pink salt
- Optional add-ins: 2 tablespoons of goji, acai, or other superfood powder

Line a 12 x 8-inch baking pan with parchment paper, leaving enough to hang over the sides. (This will help wrap and cover the top when you refrigerate the bars.)

In a large bowl, combine the hemp hearts, flaxseed, and chia seeds with the water. Allow the mixture to sit and soak up the water for about 5 minutes, until thick. Set aside.

Put the dates, goji berries, pumpkin seeds, figs, cacao nibs, chocolate chips, salt, and superfood powder (if using) in a food processor. Process on high for 20 to 30 seconds. It will be ground up and sticky.

Add the date mixture to the soaked seeds and use both hands to thoroughly mix all the ingredients together. It will be sticky and heavy, but worth all the effort!

Transfer the mixture to your prepared pan and press down evenly. Cover the bars with the overlay of parchment paper and put them in the refrigerator for about an hour.

Cut into squares and store in the refrigerator or freezer.

ANYTIME BARS
MAKES 16 BARS

I would call this snack a mix between cake and a brownie. This moist, chewy treat provides exceptional nutrients, vitamins, and much-needed minerals. Molasses adds an element of deep, robust flavor that is warm, satisfying, and nutrient dense. Flaxseed and hemp hearts act as binders and receive high marks for fiber, protein, and alpha-linoleic acid. ALA is an omega-3 fatty acid that the body cannot synthesize on its own. This fatty acid has solid antioxidant properties that aid in reducing inflammation and boosting skin structure. It is also responsible for promoting healthy nerve function and slowing the progression of memory loss disorders.

Replacing the chewy raisins with different dried fruits, cacao nibs, or dark chocolate chips would certainly be delicious!

- 3 tablespoons ground flaxseed
- 2 tablespoons hemp hearts
- 1 cup applesauce
- ⅓ cup blackstrap molasses
- ⅓ cup maple syrup
- ¼ cup coconut oil, melted
- 1½ cups gluten-free baking flour blend (I like Bob's Red Mill)

- ½ cup buckwheat flour
- 2 tablespoons cacao powder
- 1 teaspoon ground ginger
- 1½ teaspoons ground cinnamon
- 1 teaspoon baking soda
- ½ teaspoon salt
- ¾ cup raisins

Preheat the oven to 350°F. Line an 8 x 8-inch baking pan with parchment paper.

In a large bowl, combine the flaxseed, hemp hearts, applesauce, molasses, maple syrup, and coconut oil and whisk to incorporate. Set aside.

In a small bowl, combine the flour blend, buckwheat flour, cacao powder, ginger, cinnamon, baking soda, and salt. Add the dry ingredients to the wet, mixing with a spatula, then fold in the raisins. Put the thick, brownie batter–like mixture in the prepared pan. I find that it helps to slightly wet the spatula to evenly spread out the sticky mixture. Bake for 25 minutes until firm to the touch and golden brown.

Store in an airtight container. They are delicious when stored in the refrigerator and can also be frozen.

VEGAN SMITTY BITES
MAKES 24 BITES

I encountered Aussie Bites years ago while shopping in Costco. They are quite tasty, with nuts, seeds, fruits, and berries, but needed an overhaul of some of the recipe ingredients. The cleaned-up recipe contains no processed sugar and is rich in omega-3s, fiber, and protein.

Buckwheat cereal has a lower glycemic index than oats and is easier to digest; it also provides more fiber and is rich in potassium, zinc, magnesium, and B vitamins. The final product can be a snack, a yogurt topping, or complement a breakfast bowl of fruit.

- 1½ cups buckwheat cereal
- 1 cup cooked quinoa
- 4 dried apricots

- ¼ cup dried cherries
- ¼ cup dried goji berries (see notes)
- 6 Medjool dates, pitted (see notes)
- ¼ cup raisins
- ¼ cup honey
- ¼ cup pistachios (see notes)
- 3 tablespoons ground flaxseed
- ¼ cup unsweetened coconut flakes
- 1 tablespoon vanilla extract
- 1 teaspoon baking soda
- ½ teaspoon salt
- ½ cup water
- 3 tablespoons coconut oil

Preheat the oven to 350°F. Prepare a mini muffin pan. (I use an oven-friendly Silpat mini muffin pan, so I don't need to grease it. If you're using a typical mini muffin pan, grease it or use liners.)

Put all the ingredients except the coconut oil in a food processor or high-speed blender and pulse for 30 seconds until the mixture comes together. Add the coconut oil (do not melt it) and pulse again for 5 to 10 seconds. Transfer the dough to a large bowl.

Form the dough into tablespoon-size balls with your hands. Fill the prepped muffin cups to the top and push down gently on the dough.

Bake for 12 to 15 minutes until golden brown. Remove from the oven and let cool. Once cooled, remove the muffins from the pan and store them in an airtight container in the refrigerator for two weeks. These can also be frozen.

NOTES: You can use any kind of dried fruit you might have, such as cranberries, blueberries, or prunes.

Medjool dates work best because they are soft. For other kinds of dates, soak for 5 minutes in warm water first.

Mix up the nuts and substitute whatever other nuts or seeds you have—sunflower seeds, pumpkin seeds, or even something like walnuts.

CONDIMENTS, SAUCES, DIPS, AND SPREADS

TACO SEASONING
MAKES ABOUT 2 TABLESPOONS

It's easy to make your own taco seasoning to use in recipes like Mexican Baked Potatoes, Mexican Rice Bowls, Vegetable Enchiladas, and others.

- 1 tablespoon chili powder
- ½ teaspoon garlic powder
- ½ teaspoon paprika
- ½ teaspoon cumin
- 1 teaspoon salt

Mix all the ingredients together in a bowl. Store in an airtight container or mason jar.

SUN-DRIED TOMATO SPREAD
MAKES ABOUT ¾ CUP

This may be the simplest recipe I have. It is great on sandwiches and toast, as a spread, or in lieu of tomato paste. If you add a good-quality oil to the finished product, it makes a great finishing sauce for grilled vegetables or fresh summer tomato slices.

Trader Joe's sells California sun-dried tomatoes in a small 3-ounce bag. I like them because they are nice and soft. You can also add some warm water to other brands to rehydrate them if they are too hard.

- 3-ounce bag sun-dried tomatoes
- 3 tablespoons olive oil

Put the tomatoes in a high-speed blender. Blend on high, adding a tablespoon of oil at a time until you achieve the consistency of a spreadable paste. If it is too runny, add more sun-dried tomatoes. If it is too thick, add a bit more oil.

BROCCOLI OR BROCCOLI RABE PESTO
MAKES ABOUT 2 CUPS

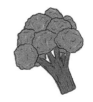

Try something different from your typical pesto on root vegetables, buckwheat noodles, pasta, pizza crust, or even wraps. Like other cruciferous vegetables, broccoli has many prominent bioactive vitamins, minerals, and antioxidants, meaning, in their natural state, these compounds are better absorbed by the body and promote good health. In addition, broccoli has impressive nutrients such as fiber and protein. It also has a more subtle taste, while broccoli rabe is more bitter and peppery. This basic pesto is a keeper worth making all year long.

- 1 head broccoli or broccoli rabe, roughly chopped, stems discarded
- ½ cup pumpkin seeds or pistachios
- 1 cup parsley
- 1 shallot, minced
- 2 cloves Roasted Garlic
- ¼ cup olive oil
- ¼ cup full-fat unsweetened canned coconut milk (optional, see note)

In a large pot, bring salted water to a boil, add the broccoli, and blanch for 3 minutes. Rinse under cold water, squeeze out excess water, and set aside.

Put the seeds in a small pan and toast lightly over medium-high heat for 4 to 5 minutes. Keep an eye on them and shake them frequently. Remove the seeds from the pan and let cool.

Put the blanched broccoli, seeds, parsley, shallot, garlic, oil, and coconut milk (if using) in a food processor. Process until well incorporated. Season with salt and pepper to taste. Keep for up to a week in the refrigerator or freeze extras for another meal.

NOTE: This recipe is fine without the coconut milk, but including it makes for an interesting creamy pesto that can be used as a finishing sauce for many dishes, such as roasted spaghetti squash.

VERDE PICO DE GALLO
MAKES ABOUT 2 CUPS

This would be great on baked potatoes, zucchini noodles, vegetarian enchiladas, or rice cakes or in a traditional dip or as a salad topper.

- 4 Persian cucumbers or 2 small cucumbers, diced
- ½ jicama, peeled and diced
- 1 avocado, diced
- 2 scallions, roughly sliced
- 1 serrano pepper, chopped, seeds removed
- 1 green bell pepper, diced
- ¼ cup pistachios or pumpkin seeds, finely chopped and toasted
- ¼ cup lime juice
- Handful of fresh cilantro, chopped
- 1 tablespoon fresh mint, chopped
- 2 tablespoons olive oil
- 1 clove Roasted Garlic, mashed into a paste

In a large bowl, combine the cucumber, jicama, avocado, scallions, serrano pepper, bell pepper, and pistachios.

In a small bowl, whisk together the lime juice, cilantro, mint, oil, and garlic paste. Fold the dressing into the chopped vegetables. Season with salt and pepper to taste.

GOLDEN BEET SALSA/SALAD
MAKES 3 CUPS

Golden beet salsa is visually gorgeous and will get those digestive enzymes flowing. It is the perfect condiment for tacos or quesadillas. I have also eaten this delicious combination as a meal, side dish, or party salad.

- 2 large or 4 medium golden beets, steamed or roasted
- 1 yellow bell pepper, diced
- 1 cup hearts of palm, diced
- ¼ cup capers
- ¼ red onion or 1 shallot, diced
- 2 tablespoons lime juice
- 2 tablespoons fresh parsley, chopped
- 2 tablespoons fresh cilantro, chopped
- 1 tablespoon coconut or apple cider vinegar
- 1 tablespoon olive oil
- 1 tablespoon fresh mint, chopped
- Pinch of chili flakes (optional)

To steam the beets, fill the bottom of a steamer with about 3 inches of water and bring to a boil. Add the beets to the steamer tray; if using larger beets, cut them in half first. Cover and steam for about 15 minutes until tender. Cool, peel, and dice.

To roast the beets, preheat the oven to 400°F. Line a baking sheet with parchment paper. Cut the beets in half (or quarters if they're on the larger side) and coat lightly with oil. Roast for 20 to 25 minutes or until the skins are soft and the beets are tender. Cool, peel, and dice.

In a large bowl, combine the diced beets, bell pepper, hearts of palm, capers, onion, lime juice, parsley, cilantro, coconut vinegar, oil, mint, and chili flakes (if using). Season with salt and pepper to taste.

SWEET ONION AND WHITE BEAN DIP
MAKES ABOUT 2 CUPS

This dip is made with white cannellini beans and takes on a completely different flavor with caramelized onions, balsamic vinegar, and capers. This dip can be used as a sandwich spread or a pizza base instead of the traditional tomato sauce. Get creative—this is a keeper.

- 1 tablespoon olive, coconut, or avocado oil
- ½ red onion, roughly chopped
- 2 garlic cloves, roughly chopped
- 1 tablespoon balsamic vinegar
- 1 (15-ounce) can white cannellini beans, well rinsed, or 2 cups home-cooked
- 2 tablespoons lemon juice, plus more to taste
- 1 teaspoon capers
- ½ teaspoon dried oregano or 1 teaspoon fresh oregano

Put the oil and onion in a saucepan and sauté over high heat for several minutes, stirring constantly. Add the garlic and continue stirring for another 3 to 5 minutes. Stir in the balsamic vinegar. Reduce the heat to low and cook for 2 to 3 minutes until the vinegar has evaporated and caramelized the onions. Remove from the heat.

Put the onion mixture, beans, lemon juice, capers, and oregano in a food processor. Process on high until smooth and creamy. Taste and add more lemon juice, if you like. Season with salt and pepper to taste.

CHILI-CARROT SPREAD
MAKES ABOUT 2 CUPS

This is a great salad dressing, condiment for a veggie burger, or base to build a quinoa or rice bowl.

- 5 to 6 carrots, shredded
- 1 shallot, diced

- 3 tablespoons orange juice
- 1 teaspoon ground cumin
- 1 teaspoon ground chili powder

Put all the ingredients in a small bowl or mason jar and whisk or shake until well combined. Season with salt and pepper to taste.

NONDAIRY CHEESY PARSNIP SAUCE
MAKES ABOUT 2 CUPS

Parsnips are one of the healthiest vegetables you can consume. This sauce is great on pasta or lasagna or with roasted vegetables (cheesy baked fries!). If you are having a party and grilling vegetables for a crowd, spread this sauce evenly on the base of your serving platter, top with roasted vegetables, and sprinkle with fresh herbs.

- 4 to 5 parsnips, chopped into 1-inch chunks (see notes)
- 1 medium white sweet potato, chopped
- 1 carrot, chopped
- 1 teaspoon Roasted Garlic
- ½ cup nutritional yeast
- ½ cup oat or other nondairy milk
- ½ teaspoon ground mustard
- 1 teaspoon ground sweet paprika
- ½ teaspoon salt
- Fresh herbs of choice (optional, see notes)

Start by steaming or boiling the vegetables.

To steam the veggies, fill the bottom of a steamer with about 3 inches of water and bring to a boil. Add the parsnips, potato, and carrot to the steamer tray. Cover and steam for about 15 minutes until tender.

To boil the veggies, bring salted water and the parsnips, potato, and carrot to a boil in a large pot. Cook until tender, 10 to 12 minutes.

Let the vegetables cool slightly and then combine them with the rest of the ingredients in a high-speed blender and blend until smooth and creamy. It's important to do this when the parsnips, potato, and carrot are warm (not hot), as this will produce a creamier mixture. I like a thick sauce, especially if I am going to use it with gluten-free pasta, but if it is too thick, you can thin it out with more milk. Season with salt and pepper to taste.

NOTES: Look for skinnier parsnips when shopping, as they are not as tough.

Depending on the dish, fresh herbs are an excellent addition. Fresh rosemary slightly roasted over a flame and pureed with the sauce would be delicious with something like roasted potatoes or a roasted vegetable platter.

ROASTED CAULIFLOWER AND BUTTERNUT SQUASH SAUCE
MAKES ABOUT 2 CUPS

This is a wonderful and versatile sauce to top pasta, lasagna (see Green Lentil Lasagna), rice, or roasted vegetables.

- 1 cup canned butternut squash puree or freshly cooked and mashed
- 1 cup cauliflower florets, roasted
- 2 cloves Roasted Garlic (see notes)
- Handful of fresh basil
- 3 tablespoons nutritional yeast
- 2 to 4 tablespoons vegetable broth
- 1 tablespoon nondairy ricotta or other nondairy cheese (I like Kite Hill and Violife, see notes)
- 1 tablespoon ground oregano
- 1 teaspoon ground turmeric

Put all the ingredients in a high-speed blender or blender cup and blend until well combined and creamy. Do not process too long or it may become too gummy. Season with salt and pepper to taste.

NOTES: If you do not have any roasted garlic, sauté garlic cloves in a little olive oil for several minutes.

If you cannot find nondairy cheese, you can substitute 1 small peeled and boiled potato and 1 more tablespoon of nutritional yeast.

ACKNOWLEDGMENTS

My health situations have required specialists, functional medicine doctors, health coaches, and probably too many Google searches. Not too long ago, as I was starting to believe that I was imagining all my ailments, one of my best learning moments came from a fellow health coach who shared her journey with me and listened to mine, helping me fine-tune my path. Knowing that you are not alone always helps. Thank you, Kristy Klymciw!

The best advice I have ever been given was by a doctor who told me to remember that I was paying him for his guidance and services, that I was the boss and should always feel comfortable in whichever way my healthcare led me. Thank you, Dr. Keith McCormick—your bedside manner and kindness are forever appreciated. I am grateful for your guidance.

I am also grateful to my ob-gyn for her kindness and support in this journey. Knowing you were there with whatever I needed provided comfort whenever a situation looked bleak. Thank you, Dr. Meg Hainer. I should also praise the functional medicine doctor that made the cut, so thank you, Dr. Douglas Pucci. Your infinite knowledge gave me so much to ponder as I learned more about what made me feel my best. Our sessions often ran quite over, as you loved to talk and I loved to listen, challenge, absorb, and understand the mind-body facet so critical to healing.

Next, a huge thank you to my book coach, Marisa Solis, for the quality time we spent outlining, editing, organizing, and shaping the book I saw in my head. My gratitude cannot be expressed enough in words. I am genuinely thankful for your leadership and confidence in my vision.

What better way to facilitate this thought bubble of a book than to enlist Girl Friday Productions to help me self-publish it. My competent team gave me complete creative control all while leading me to the best version of my personal vision. Thank you to Christina Henry de Tessan, Sara Spees Addicott, Audra Figgins, Heena Aswani, Adria Batt, and Paul Barrett.

Last, but not least, a huge thank you to Erin Hart, my sweet, adorable, and exceptionally talented illustrator. Though she is a whole generation younger than me, she is so in tune with my vision as someone who has struggled with her own health issues. She is my mini-me when it comes to wanting the most robust outcome with food, health, and the mind-body connection. Erin, I appreciate your drive, time, and passion.

You're on the list too, Smitty. Now I can get out of the house more. Thank you for your continued love and support.

DIRTY DOZEN AND CLEAN FIFTEEN FOODS

The Dirty Dozen

The fruits and veggies with the MOST pesticide residue

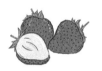

Strawberries

Spinach

Celery

Nectarines

Apples

Grapes

Cherries

Peaches

Pears

Bell & Hot Peppers

Kale, Collard & Mustard Greens

Tomatoes

The Clean Fifteen

The fruits and veggies with the **LEAST** pesticide residue

Avocados

Sweet Corn

Pineapples

Onions

Papayas

Sweet Peas

Eggplants

Asparagus

Cabbage

Kiwis

Cauliflower

Mushrooms

Broccoli

Honeydew Melon

Cantaloupe

RESET 90/10
MENU SUGGESTIONS

Sample Menu: Week 1

	Breakfast	Snack	Lunch	Dinner	Snack
Monday	Celery juice (wait 20 min.) Warm lemon water (wait 20 min.) Energy fruit smoothie	Fresh fruit	Salad bowl w/ roasted vegetables	Spaghetti squash w/ nondairy cheese sauce Simple salad	Pumpkin buckwheat cereal muffin
Tuesday	Celery juice (wait 20 min.) Warm lemon water (wait 20 min.) Energy fruit smoothie	Fresh fruit	Spaghetti squash leftovers Simple salad	Tomato, fennel, and sweet potato soup	Seaweed snacks
Wednesday	Celery juice (wait 20 min.) Warm lemon water (wait 20 min.) Energy fruit smoothie	Fresh fruit	Leftover tomato-fennel soup w/ quinoa Simple salad	Simply mashed Simple salad w/ olives	Dried fruit
Thursday	Celery juice (wait 20 min.) Warm lemon water (wait 20 min.) Energy fruit smoothie	Fresh fruit	Roasted spiralized vegetables Simple salad	Leftover roasted spiralized vegetables w/ buckwheat noodles & whipped tahini sauce	Applesauce w/ dried mulberries
Friday	Celery juice (wait 20 min.) Warm lemon water (wait 20 min.) Energy fruit smoothie	Fresh fruit	Green pea falafel w/ orange-tahini herb sauce over a simple salad	Collard green wrap w/ green pea falafel and steamed asparagus	Dates and tahini w/ raw honey
Saturday	Celery juice (wait 20 min.) Warm lemon water (wait 20 min.) Energy fruit smoothie	Fresh fruit	Buckwheat pancakes	Baked sweet potato w/ whipped tahini sauce & steamed asparagus Simple salad	Dried mulberries
Sunday	Celery juice (wait 20 min.) Warm lemon water (wait 20 min.) Energy fruit smoothie	Fresh fruit	Baked potato fries w/ half an avocado & steamed green beans	Ginger pumpkin soup (freeze leftovers for next week) Simple salad	Baked potato chips w/ beet salsa

Sample Menu: Week 2

	Breakfast	Snack	Lunch	Dinner	Snack
Monday	Celery juice (wait 20 min.) Warm lemon water (wait 20 min.) Energy fruit smoothie	Fresh fruit	English method of roasting potatoes and carrots, w/ yuzu pea puree	Roasted sweet potato fried rice w/ sliced avocado & cilantro-lime sauce Simple salad	Frozen banana cream
Tuesday	Celery juice (wait 20 min.) Warm lemon water (wait 20 min.) Energy fruit smoothie	Fresh fruit	English potato leftovers w/ cilantro-lime sauce Simple salad	Roasted sweet potato fried rice salad bowl w/ green goddess vinaigrette	Dried figs
Wednesday	Celery juice (wait 20 min.) Warm lemon water (wait 20 min.) Energy fruit smoothie	Fresh fruit	Leftover ginger pumpkin soup (from freezer)	Vegetable sushi roll (takeout) Simple salad w/ simple salad vinaigrette	Rice cake with beet salsa
Thursday	Celery juice (wait 20 min.) Warm lemon water (wait 20 min.) Energy fruit smoothie	Fresh fruit	Savory vegetable cakes w/ pickled radish & half an avocado	Tomato, fennel, and sweet potato soup w/ rice (freeze leftovers for next week)	Dates and tahini
Friday	Celery juice (wait 20 min.) Warm lemon water (wait 20 min.) Energy fruit smoothie	Fresh fruit	Baked sweet potato w/ avocado, salsa, and cilantro-lime sauce Simple salad	Collard green wrap w/ savory vegetable cakes & tahini dipping sauce Peeled cucumber salad	Buckwheat pancakes w/ maple syrup
Saturday	Celery juice (wait 20 min.) Warm lemon water (wait 20 min.) Energy fruit smoothie	Fresh fruit	Buddha bowl with quinoa and spiralized squash	Hearty vegetable soup Simple salad	Goji berries mixed with dried mulberries
Sunday	Celery juice (wait 20 min.) Warm lemon water (wait 20 min.) Energy fruit smoothie	Fresh fruit	Leftover hearty vegetable soup w/ rice	Raw pad thai noodle salad	Dried apricots

Sample Menu: Week 3

	Breakfast	Snack	Lunch	Dinner	Snack
Monday	Celery juice (wait 20 min.) Warm lemon water (wait 20 min.) Energy fruit smoothie	Fresh fruit	Leftover raw pad thai noodle salad	Simply mashed w/ green peas Simple salad	Pumpkin buckwheat cereal muffin w/ a touch of maple syrup
Tuesday	Celery juice (wait 20 min.) Warm lemon water (wait 20 min.) Energy fruit smoothie	Fresh fruit	Cream of buckwheat cereal w/ quick applesauce	Green pea falafel w/ orange-tahini herb sauce & baked potato	Dates and tahini
Wednesday	Celery juice (wait 20 min.) Warm lemon water (wait 20 min.) Energy fruit smoothie	Fresh fruit	Buckwheat and roasted vegetable tabbouleh salad	Savory vegetable cakes w/ yuzu pea puree & olives Simple salad	Dried mango slices
Thursday	Celery juice (wait 20 min.) Warm lemon water (wait 20 min.) Energy fruit smoothie	Fresh fruit	Roasted vegetables w/ nondairy cheese sauce	Leftover buckwheat and roasted vegetable tabbouleh salad w/ green pea falafel	Quick applesauce & dried mulberries
Friday	Celery juice (wait 20 min.) Warm lemon water (wait 20 min.) Energy fruit smoothie	Fresh fruit	Tomato, fennel, and sweet potato soup (from freezer) w/ quinoa	Roasted vegetables w/ tahini dressing Simple salad	Frozen banana cream
Saturday	Celery juice (wait 20 min.) Warm lemon water (wait 20 min.) Energy fruit smoothie	Fresh fruit	Sautéed vegetables w/ mixed herb pesto & quinoa	Roasted butternut squash, purple potatoes & artichokes hearts Simple salad	Seaweed snacks
Sunday	Celery juice (wait 20 min.) Warm lemon water (wait 20 min.) Energy fruit smoothie	Fresh fruit	Savory vegetable cakes w/ quick pickled radish, diced cooked beets, and olives	Leftover sautéed vegetables w/ mixed herb pesto and ½ of a roasted acorn squash	Dried mulberries

BLANK MENU

You can also download a blank menu planner at www.chefellen.com.

	Breakfast	Snack	Lunch	Dinner	Snack
Monday					
Tuesday					
Wednesday					
Thursday					
Friday					
Saturday					
Sunday					

FOOD AND
SYMPTOM TRACKER

This is a convenient way to record reintroduced foods to accurately monitor foods that may cause discomfort. Making the connection between symptoms and the food you are taking in is a useful and effective way to organize any dietary changes as you go through Reset and Maintenance.

Today's Food and Symptom Tracker

	Food/Drink	Symptoms	Bowel Movement	Triggers
Breakfast				
Snack				
Lunch				
Dinner				
Snack				

TODAY'S FOOD REINTRODUCTION

Food	👍	👎	Retry

NOTES

TODAY'S WATER INTAKE

◊ ◊ ◊ ◊ ◊ ◊ ◊ ◊ ◊ ◊ ◊ ◊ ◊ ◊ ◊

1 droplet = 8 ounces

TODAY'S MOOD

 ecstatic   happy   okay   moody   unhappy   very sad

TODAY'S POOP TYPE

 constipation *(severe)*   constipation *(mild)*   normal   normal   lacking fiber   diarrhea *(mild)*   diarrhea *(severe)*

TODAY'S PAIN LEVEL

 no pain   mild   moderate   painful   horrible   unbearable

NOTES

1   https://www.nationaleatingdisorders.org/learn/by-eating-disorder
    /anorexia
2   https://www.integrativenutrition.com/dietarytheories
3   https://thenutritionalinstitute.com/resources/blog/292-the-4-r-s-of-gut
    -health
4   https://med.libretexts.org/Courses/American_Public_University/
    APU%3A_Basic_Foundation_of_Nutrition_for_Sports_Performance
    _(Byerley)/03%3A_Digestion_and_Absorption/3.3%3A_The_Digestion
    _and_Absorption_Process
5   https://www.ncbi.nlm.nih.gov/books/NBK279304/
6   https://www.niddk.nih.gov/health-information/digestive-diseases
    /digestive-system-how-it-works
7   https://fadavispt.mhmedical.com/content.aspx?bookid=2641&sectionid
    =217178679
8   https://www.heartuk.org.uk/downloads/health-professionals/publications
    /blood-fats-explained.pdf
9   https://www.ncbi.nlm.nih.gov/pmc/articles/PMC4838534/
10 https://www.health.harvard.edu/blog/diet-and-depression
    -2018022213309
11 https://www.ncbi.nlm.nih.gov/pmc/articles/PMC7284805/
12 https://pubmed.ncbi.nlm.nih.gov/31071306/
13 https://www.ncbi.nlm.nih.gov/pmc/articles/PMC6790068/
14 https://medlineplus.gov/ency/article/000816.htm
15 https://www.ncbi.nlm.nih.gov/pmc/articles/PMC1856434/
16 https://www.mayoclinic.org/tests-procedures/stool-dna-test/about
    /pac-20385153
17 https://www.mentalhelp.net/health-policy-and-advocacy/being-an
    -effective-self-advocate/
    https://health.usnews.com/health-news/patient-advice/articles/2015/02
    /02/6-ways-to-be-your-own-health-advocate

18 https://www.news-medical.net/news/20200611/Nutritional-study
    -shows-wide-range-of-metabolic-responses-after-eating-in-healthy
    -adults.aspx

19 https://www.ncbi.nlm.nih.gov/pmc/articles/PMC3959903/#:~:text=
    Alcohol%20is%20highly%20diffusible%20through,for%20alcohol
    %2Dinduced%20organ%20damage

20 https://drhyman.com/blog/2012/06/13/ten-reasons-to-quit-your-coffee/

21 https://www.tandfonline.com/doi/full/10.1080/10408398.2014.967385

22 https://www.ncbi.nlm.nih.gov/pmc/articles/PMC4586567/

23 https://www.epa.gov/mercury/how-people-are-exposed-mercury

24 https://link.springer.com/article/10.1007/s11356-021-18110-0#:~:text
    =Glyphosate%20is%20detected%20in%2099.8,equal%20to%200.0%20ng
    %2Fml

25 https://wwwn.cdc.gov/Nchs/Nhanes/2013-2014/SSGLYP_H.htm

26 https://pubmed.ncbi.nlm.nih.gov/29216767/
    https://www.ncbi.nlm.nih.gov/pmc/articles/PMC3945755

27 https://www.imrpress.com/journal/FBL/23/12/10.2741/4704

28 https://pubmed.ncbi.nlm.nih.gov/20536509/

29 https://www.ncbi.nlm.nih.gov/pmc/articles/PMC7231027/

30 https://www.ncbi.nlm.nih.gov/pmc/articles/PMC6124841/

31 https://www.dietaryguidelines.gov/sites/default/files/2020-12/Dietary
    _Guidelines_for_Americans_2020-2025.pdf

32 https://www.researchgate.net/figure/Comparison-of-rationale-evidence
    -and-dietary-restrictions-in-published-diets-aimed-at_tbl2_236184858

33 https://www.thelancet.com/journals/ebiom/article/PIIS2352
    -3964(21)00086-4/fulltext

34 https://www.ncbi.nlm.nih.gov/pmc/articles/PMC3735932/

35 https://www.ncbi.nlm.nih.gov/pmc/articles/PMC6389125/

36 https://microbiomejournal.biomedcentral.com/articles/10.1186/s40168
    -020-00875-0
    https://drhyman.com/blog/2012/06/13/ten-reasons-to-quit-your-coffee/

37 https://atlasbiomed.com/blog/whats-the-difference-between-microbiome
    -and-microbiota/#microbiome-microbiota

38 https://bmjopen.bmj.com/content/6/3/e009892
    https://pubmed.ncbi.nlm.nih.gov/18042305/

39 https://www.sciencedirect.com/science/article/abs/pii/
    S0140673668909082

https://www.health.harvard.edu/blog/nutritional-psychiatry-your-brain
-on-food-201511168626

40 https://www.integrativenutrition.com/blog/what-does-a-health-coach-do

41 https://www.simplypsychology.org/fight-flight-freeze-fawn.html

42 https://link.springer.com/article/10.1007/BF03345606

43 https://www.integrativenutrition.com/blog/2008/03/26/primary-food

44 https://www.scientificamerican.com/article/gut-second-brain/

45 https://www.hopkinsmedicine.org/research/advancements-in-research
/fundamentals/in-depth/the-gut-where-bacteria-and-immune-system
-meet

46 https://www.health.harvard.edu/blog/diet-and-depression-
2018022213309

47 https://pubmed.ncbi.nlm.nih.gov/33693453

48 https://pubmed.ncbi.nlm.nih.gov/34277527/

49 https://www.ncbi.nlm.nih.gov/pmc/articles/PMC7692600
https://www.hopkinsmedicine.org/research/advancements-in-research
/fundamentals/in-depth/the-gut-where-bacteria-and-immune-system-meet

50 https://www.frontiersin.org/articles/10.3389/fpsyt.2018.00044/full

51 https://pubmed.ncbi.nlm.nih.gov/32572435/

52 https://pubmed.ncbi.nlm.nih.gov/27988382/
https://neuroscience.ubc.ca/our-second-brain-more-than-a-gut-feeling/

53 https://www.frontiersin.org/articles/10.3389/fmed.2018.00053/full

54 https://www.healthline.com/human-body-maps/pituitary-gland#1
https://neuroscientificallychallenged.com/posts/what-is-the-hpa-axis

55 https://www.niddk.nih.gov/health-information/diabetes/overview/
what-is-diabetes/prediabetes-insulin-resistance

56 https://www.ncbi.nlm.nih.gov/pmc/articles/PMC6710489/

57 https://www.apa.org/topics/stress/body

58 https://www.neuroscientificallychallenged.com/blog/2014/5/31/what-is
-the-hpa-axis
https://www.integrativenutrition.com/dietarytheories

59 https://www.cell.com/neuron/fulltext/S0896-6273(12)00941-5?
_returnURL=https%3A%2F%2Flinkinghub.elsevier.com%2Fretrieve
%2Fpii%2FS0896627312009415%3Fshowall%3Dtrue

60 https://www.nature.com/articles/npre.2009.3790.1

61 https://www.gutmicrobiotaforhealth.com/scientists-identified-two
-bacteria-from-gut-microbiota-linked-to-mental-health/

62 https://www.health.harvard.edu/blog/when-dieting-doesnt-work
    -2020052519889

63 https://www.health.harvard.edu/nutrition/when-it-comes-to-protein
    -how-much-is-too-much
    https://www.cdc.gov/nchs/fastats/diet.htm

64 https://www.cedars-sinai.org/blog/best-protein.html

65 https://www.ncbi.nlm.nih.gov/pmc/articles/PMC4332360/

66 https://www.acpjournals.org/doi/full/10.7326/M19-1326

67 https://www.ncbi.nlm.nih.gov/pmc/articles/PMC4991651/

68 https://pubmed.ncbi.nlm.nih.gov/28701046/

69 https://www.medicalnewstoday.com/articles/324932#summary

70 https://www.medicalnewstoday.com/articles/321993

71 https://www.ncbi.nlm.nih.gov/pmc/articles/PMC3249911/

72 https://pubmed.ncbi.nlm.nih.gov/11354540/

73 https://www.ncbi.nlm.nih.gov/pmc/articles/PMC5871295/

74 https://www.ncbi.nlm.nih.gov/pmc/articles/PMC6363527/
    https://microbiomejournal.biomedcentral.com/articles/10.1186/s40168
    -020-00875-0

75 https://www.ncbi.nlm.nih.gov/pmc/articles/PMC3436979/

76 https://www.purdue.edu/uns/html4ever/1997/9712.Savaiano.intolerance
    .html

77 https://www.ncbi.nlm.nih.gov/pmc/articles/PMC5004213/

78 https://www.ncbi.nlm.nih.gov/pmc/articles/PMC6790068/

79 https://www.ncbi.nlm.nih.gov/pmc/articles/PMC4716040/
    https://www.ncbi.nlm.nih.gov/pmc/articles/PMC6389125/

80 https://www.researchgate.net/publication/333912508_Crohn's_Disease
    _Remission_with_a_Plant-Based_Diet_A_Case_Report

81 https://www.testing.com/tests/thyroid-antibodies/

82 https://www.beyondceliac.org/gluten-free-diet/common-food-safety
    -questions/food-safety-what-is-glyphosate-and-what-does-it-have-to-do
    -with-celiac-disease/

83 https://www.ncbi.nlm.nih.gov/pmc/articles/PMC6790068/#R6

84 https://www.sciencedirect.com/science/article/pii/S2214750018300362
    https://www.ncbi.nlm.nih.gov/pmc/articles/PMC1856434/

85 https://www.sciencedirect.com/science/article/pii/S2214750018300362
    https://www.healthline.com/human-body-maps/pituitary-gland#1

86 https://www.nature.com/articles/nature13793

87   https://www.ncbi.nlm.nih.gov/pmc/articles/PMC1931610/
88   https://www.ncbi.nlm.nih.gov/pmc/articles/PMC5405737/
     https://www.ncbi.nlm.nih.gov/pmc/articles/PMC5617129/
89   https://www.ncbi.nlm.nih.gov/pmc/articles/PMC7600777/
90   https://branchbasics.com/blogs/food/do-you-have-enough-hcl-stomach
     -acid?_pos=1&_sid=2b9f3dca3&_ss=r
91   https://www.ncbi.nlm.nih.gov/pmc/articles/PMC6723943/
92   https://www.ncbi.nlm.nih.gov/books/NBK554493/
93   https://www.webmd.com/allergies/what-are-histamines
94   https://www.ncbi.nlm.nih.gov/pmc/articles/PMC7468712/
95   https://pubmed.ncbi.nlm.nih.gov/24533607/
96   https://www.ncbi.nlm.nih.gov/pmc/articles/PMC6138814/#:~:text
     =The%20link%20between%20oxidative%20stress,even%20late%20stage
     %20diabetes%20cases
97   https://pubmed.ncbi.nlm.nih.gov/18346005/
98   https://pubmed.ncbi.nlm.nih.gov/9408743/
99   https://www.niddk.nih.gov/health-information/digestive-diseases/acid
     -reflux-ger-gerd-adults
     https://www.healthline.com/health/gerd
100 https://www.ncbi.nlm.nih.gov/pmc/articles/PMC6862638/
101 https://www.mayoclinic.org/chronic-pain-medication-decisions/art
     -20360371
102 https://www.medicalnewstoday.com/articles/310215#pain-management
     -plans

RESOURCES

BOOKS AND ARTICLES

GENERAL HEALTH

"6 Ways to Be Your Own Health Advocate" by Elizabeth Renter, health. usnews.com/health-news/patient-advice/articles/2015/02/02/6 -ways-to-be-your-own-health-advocate

How to Be Well: The 6 Keys to a Happy and Healthy Life by Frank Lipman, MD

The Immune System Recovery Plan: A Doctor's 4-Step Plan by Susan Blum, MD, MPH

UnDo It!: How Simple Lifestyle Changes Can Reverse Most Chronic Diseases by Dean Ornish, MD, and Anne Ornish

The Unmaking of a Drug Dealer: A Physician's Journey to Find Truth by Patricia Hopkins, MD

Your Body in Balance: The New Science of Food, Hormones, and Health by Neal D. Barnard, MD, FACC

FOOD AND COOKBOOKS

Eat to Live Quick and Easy Cookbook: 131 Delicious Recipes for Fast and Sustained Weight Loss, Reversing Disease, and Lifelong Health by Joel Fuhrman, MD

"Impact of Dietary Fat on Gut Microbiota and Low-Grade Systemic

Inflammation: Mechanisms and Clinical Implications on Obesity" in *International Journal of Food Sciences and Nutrition* by Flávia Galvão Cândido et al., pubmed.ncbi.nlm.nih.gov/28675945/

I Quit Sugar: Your Complete 8-Week Detox Program and Cookbook by Sarah Wilson

It's Just Personal: A Personal Chef's Essential Guide to Shopping, Cooking, and Eating Smarter by Ellen Postolowski

Seven Countries Study, Ancel Keys et al., www.sevencountriesstudy.com

"The Effects of Diet on Inflammation: Emphasis on the Metabolic Syndrome" in *Journal of the American College of Cardiology* by Dario Giugliano, Antonio Ceriello, and Katherine Esposito, pubmed.ncbi.nlm.nih.gov/16904534/

The Food Babe Way: Break Free from the Hidden Toxins in Your Food and Lose Weight, Look Years Younger, and Get Healthy in Just 21 Days! by Vani Hari

The Low Carb Myth: Free Yourself from Carb Myths, and Discover the Secret Keys That Really Determine Your Health and Fat Loss Destiny by Ari Whitten and Wade Smith, MD

The Plant-Based Diet Revolution: 28 Days to a Happier Gut and a Healthier You by Dr. Alan Desmond

The Plant-Based Solution: America's Healthy Heart Doc's Plan to Power Your Health by Joel K. Kahn, MD

The Proof Is in the Plants: How Science Shows a Plant-Based Diet Could Save Your Life by Simon Hill

MENTAL HEALTH

Conversations with the Goddesses: Revealing the Divine Power Within You by Agapi Stassinopoulos

"Inner Smile Meditation" by Lee Holden, youtube.com/watch?v=lLu7X7flE5U

Living an Uncommon Life: Essential Lessons From 21 Extraordinary People by John St. Augustine

Positively Resilient: 5½ Secrets to Beat Stress, Overcome Obstacles, and Defeat Anxiety by Doug Hensch

The Gifts of Imperfection: Let Go of Who You Think You're Supposed to Be and Embrace Who You Are by Brené Brown, PhD, MSW

"3 Effective Ways to Advocate for Yourself in the Workplace" by Kwame
    Christian, forbes.com/sites/kwamechristian/2021/03/31/3-effective
    -ways-to-advocate-for-yourself-in-the-workplace/?sh=7e1854592061
"What Is Self-Advocacy?" by Andrew M. I. Lee, JD, understood.org
    /en/articles/the-importance-of-self-advocacy

SPECIFIC ISSUES

*Chronic: The Hidden Cause of the Autoimmune Pandemic and How to
    Get Healthy Again* by Steven Phillips, MD, and Dana Parish, with
    Kristin Loberg
"How People Are Exposed to Mercury" by United States Environmental
    Protection Agency, epa.gov/mercury/how-people-are-exposed
    -mercury
*Medical Medium Cleanse to Heal: Healing Plans for Sufferers of
    Anxiety, Depression, Acne, Eczema, Lyme, Gut Problems, Brain
    Fog, Weight Issues, Migraines, Bloating, Vertigo, Psoriasis, Cysts,
    Fatigue, PCOS, Fibroids, UTI, Endometriosis, and Autoimmune* by
    Anthony William
*New Menopausal Years: The Wise Woman Way, Alternative Approaches
    for Women 30–90* by Susun S. Weed
Osteoporosis: An Exercise Guide by Margie Bissinger, MS, PT
*The Wisdom of Menopause: Creating Physical and Emotional Health
    During the Change* by Christiane Northrup, MD
*The Whole-Body Approach to Osteoporosis: How to Improve Bone
    Strength and Reduce Your Fracture Risk* by R. Keith McCormick, DC
*What's Missing from Medicine: Six Lifestyle Changes to Overcome
    Chronic Illness* by Saray Stancic, MD

CENTERS AND PROFESSIONALS

Dr. Douglas J. Pucci, DC, FAAIM, Functional Medicine, Neurology,
    and Nutrition, drdougpucci.com
IIN Institute for Integrative Nutrition, integrativenutrition.com
National Institute of Arthritis and Musculoskeletal and Skin Diseases,
    Osteoporosis and Related Bone Diseases National Resource
    Center, bones.nih.gov

PRODUCTS

ACCESSORIES

Souper Cubes, soupercubes.com

CANNED GOODS

Farmer's Market, farmersmarketfoods.com

COCONUT WATER

Harmless Harvest, harmlessharvest.com

CONDIMENTS AND SEASONINGS

Frontier Co-Op, frontiercoop.com
Maine Coast Sea Seasonings, seaveg.com
Mrs. Dash, mrsdash.com
Primal Kitchen, primalkitchen.com
Red Clay Hot Sauce, redclayhotsauce.com
Red Duck Foods, redduckfoods.com
Roland, rolandfoods.com
The Dandelion Kitchen, dandelionkitchen.biz

DRIED FRUITS

Natural Delights, naturaldelights.com
Sunny Fruit, sunnyfruit.com

FLOURS, GRAINS, AND BAKED GOODS

Anthony's Goods, anthonysgoods.com
Bob's Red Mill, bobsredmill.com
GluteNull, glutenull.com
Lovebird Foods, lovebirdfoods.com
One Degree Organic Foods, onedegreeorganics.com

Simple Kneads, simplekneads.com

GENERAL

Auga, augaorganics.com
Brad's Organic, bradsorganic.com
Eden, store.edenfoods.com
Food for Life, foodforlife.com
Navitas Organics, navitasorganics.com
Spectrum, spectrumbrands.com
True Elements, true-elements.com
Woodstock, woodstock-foods.com

HEMP

Manitoba Harvest, manitobaharvest.com

MEXICAN CUISINE

Frontera Foods, fronterafoods.com
Siete Family Foods, sietefoods.com

NUT BUTTERS

Artisana Organics, artisanaorganics.com
Nutiva, nutiva.com

PLANT-BASED PASTA

Big Green Organic Food, biggreenorganic.com
Chickapea, chickapea.com
Explore Cuisine, explorecuisine.com
King Soba, kingsoba.com

PLANT-BASED DAIRY

Elmhurst 1925, elmhurst1925.com

Forager Project, foragerproject.com
Lavva, lovvelavva.com
Malk, malkorganics.com
Nancy's, nancysyogurt.com
Three Trees, threetrees.com
Willa's Kitchen, willaskitchen.com

RICE

Lotus Foods, lotusfoods.com
Natural Heaven, eatnaturalheaven.com

SNACKS AND QUICK MEALS

Annie's, annies.com
Amy's, amys.com
Cascadian Farm, cascadianfarm.com
Go Raw, goraw.com
Love Beets, lovebeets.com
Lundberg, lundberg.com
Nature's Path, naturespath.com
SeaSnax, seasnax.com
Truvani, truvani.com

SOUP MIXES

Anderson House, andersonhousefoods.com

SUPPLEMENTS

Garden of Life, gardenoflife.com
Naked Seed, nakednutrition.com
Sprout Living, sproutliving.com
Sunfood Superfoods, sunfood.com

ABOUT THE AUTHOR

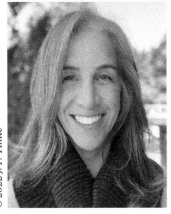

Ellen Postolowski has spent most of her career assisting clients with the changes needed to succeed in establishing a healthier lifestyle. Her work as a health-minded chef, and her complementary integrative nutrition training, honed her focus on educating and coaching people to make choices that support their health both on and off the plate. She is passionate about using her platform to change today's world of rampant auto-immune diseases, magic pills, cure-alls, fad diets, weight-image stigmas, and the stress associated with all of the above. The mind-body connection is just as important as the food on your plate.

Postolowski's back-to-basics approach of balance, awareness, and education focuses on client individuality in order to help them look, feel, and live their best lives possible.

She holds a culinary degree from the Auguste Escoffier School of Culinary Arts in Boulder, Colorado, and is a certified health coach with multiple certifications in gut and hormonal health. Postolowski lives with her family in Allendale, New Jersey, where she continues to change the lives and habits of many people looking for positive shifts and balance.

Follow her at www.chefellen.com, @chefellen on Instagram, and @iamgutdriven on TikTok for news and contact information.

CPSIA information can be obtained
at www.ICGtesting.com
Printed in the USA
BVHW052110070223
658071BV00011B/253